Resident's Guide To Starting In Medical Practice

Resident's Guide To Starting In Medical Practice

edited by

C. James Holliman, M.D., F.A.C.E.P.

Associate Professor of Surgery and Emergency Medicine
Associate Program Director, York-Hershey Emergency Medicine Residency Program
Education Coordinator and Director of the Center for International Emergency Medicine
M.S. Hershey Medical Center
Pennsylvania State University School of Medicine
Hershey, Pennsylvania

SANS TACHE

Williams & Wilkins

BALTIMORE • PHILADELPHIA • HONG KONG
LONDON • MUNICH • SYDNEY • TOKYO

A WAVERLY COMPANY

Editor: David C. Retford
Managing Editor: Kathleen Courtney Millet
Production Coordinator: Anne G. Seitz
Copy Editors: Shelley Potler, Bonnie Cover
Designer: Dan Pfisterer
Illustration Planner: Ray Lowman

Williams & Wilkins
428 East Preston Street
Baltimore, Maryland 21202 USA

Accurate indications, adverse reactions, and dosage schedules for drugs are provided in this book, but it is possible that they may change. The reader is urged to review the package information data of the manufacturers of the medications mentioned.

Printed in the United States of America

Library of Congress Cataloging-in-Publication Data

Residents guide to starting in medical practice / edited by C. James Holliman.
p. cm.
Includes bibliographical references and index.
ISBN 0-683-04125-8
1. Medicine—Practice. 2. Residents (Medicine) I. Holliman, C. James.
[DNLM: 1. Practice Management, Medical—organization & administration.
2. Private Practice—organization & administration.
W 89 R433 1995]
R728.R47 1995
610′.68—dc20
DNLM/DLC
for Library of Congress

94-36733
CIP

1 2 3 4 5 6 7 8 9 10
95 96 97 98 99

Preface

The idea for writing this book came from interaction with residents of different specialties and their common complaint of never receiving any significant advice or training regarding the nonmedical aspects of starting in medical practice after residency. Resident physicians at many academic training institutions do not receive any formal instruction on the business aspects of medical practice or on other practical aspects of medical career development. As a faculty member at an academic teaching institution, I am in the business of encouraging residents and medical students to go into academic or research-oriented medical careers. However, about half of the residents in all specialties, even at academic institutions, choose private practice for their careers. I believe that it is a responsibility of the training institution to provide instruction on career development choices as well as the paperwork and business aspects of medical practice to satisfy the needs of the relatively large number of residents who will be entering private practice.

The goals of this book are to:

1. Provide a detailed but readable reference on the important nonclinical items involved in starting private medical practice.
2. Help residents develop a planned timetable for their last year of residency to ensure that they are ready to start private practice as soon as their residency is completed.
3. Help residents avoid legal entanglements as they enter private practice.
4. Condense the information available from other sources on private practice into a format that is actually affordable by residents.

It is anticipated that residents who plan to enter academic medical practice will also find this book useful. The information in the book on choosing a community, writing a CV, and interviewing skills are all certainly important in starting an academic career and not just for residents planning on private practice.

Although most of the information presented in this book is available from other sources, a resident could expend a very large amount of money buying all the publications currently available that cover the same spread of information as presented in this book. Each chapter in the book covers the same material as is commonly presented in a single separate publication available from other sources. (These other sources are listed in Chapter 14.) The authors have experience in both private practice and in academic medical practice and hope that the book will be a useful resource for residents in planning their careers.

The chapters of the book are presented in the general order that different items need to be considered or addressed when going into private practice. Chapter 5 contains a specific recommended timetable for scheduling items during the last year of residency in preparation for private practice.

Every effort has been made to make the book as up-to-date as possible, although new laws and regulations passed since the writing of the book may alter some of the information presented.

I hope you will enjoy this book and find it useful and would welcome any criticisms or suggestions for a second edition.

C. James Holliman, M.D., FACEP

Acknowledgments

I would like to thank Donna Rentzel for her tireless efforts at typing, retyping, and editing the manuscript for this book.

I would like to thank my wife, Karen, for her patience in tolerating the 75- to 80-hour work weeks required to put this book together.

Legal Disclaimer

This book is not intended or written as a substitute for professional legal advice. The information in the book is presented in such fashion as to be applicable to the majority of situations, but may not be correct for every particular situation. Readers are advised to consult an attorney for legal advice when a situation may be different than the broadly described situations in this book.

Contributors

MEDICAL CONTRIBUTORS

David A. DeHart, M.D., F.A.C.E.P.
Senior Faculty, University of Pittsburgh
Affiliated Residency in Emergency Medicine
Past Chairman, Department of Emergency Medicine, West Penn Hospital
Member, Practice Management Committee of the American College of Emergency Physicians
President, Three Rivers Physician Service
Pittsburgh, Pennsylvania

George L. Ellis, M.D., F.A.C.E.P.
Emergency Medicine
Guthrie Clinic/Robert Packer Hospital
Sayre, Pennsylvania

H. Arnold Muller, M.D., F.A.C.E.P.
Professor of Emergency Medicine
M.S. Hershey Medical Center
Pennsylvania State University School of Medicine
Hershey, Pennsylvania
Chief of Staff
Veterans Administration Hospital
Lebanon, Pennsylvania

Richard C. Wuerz, M.D.
Assistant Professor of Emergency Medicine
Associate Director for Prehospital and Flight Services
M.S. Hershey Medical Center
Pennsylvania State University School of Medicine
Hershey, Pennsylvania

EDITORIAL ASSOCIATE

Donna J. Rentzel
Center for Emergency Medicine
M.S. Hershey Medical Center
Hershey, Pennsylvania

Contents

Chapter 1

Choosing Private Practice Versus Other Career Options

GOALS

The goals of this chapter are to point out the advantages and disadvantages of different forms of medical practice, and provide a reference list of initial contacts to investigate for medical positions.

INTRODUCTION

There are a wide range of career options available to you as graduating resident physicians. To allow sufficient time for decision-making, you should begin to solidify your postresidency career choices about halfway through residency. The general process of initiating a solo medical practice or interviewing with an existing practice, hospital, or managed care group usually requires approximately 6 months, including paperwork completion and other preparatory items. However, allowing yourself longer than 6 months will allow greater flexibility in arranging a postresidency career.

Consider taking a 1- or 2-month vacation between graduation from residency and entering private practice, if your time and finances allow. Unfortunately, large student loans or career/contractual obligations may prevent such a vacation. Even on a limited budget, it can be relatively inexpensive to go on a long car trip around the country (especially if you can stay with friends or relatives). Such a trip may be partially tax deductible if you use some of it to look for a place to live or have any formal work interview appointments. Realistically, this may be the last available chance you have for a vacation of this length for a number of years.

Postresidency career options are listed in Table 1.1. The relative advantages and disadvantages of each will subsequently be discussed in this chapter.

PRIVATE PRACTICE

As demonstrated in Table 1.1, there are a number of options for career opportunities in private medical practice. The main choices within private practice are (*a*) solo practice versus joining a group and (*b*) buying a practice (or "buying into" a practice) versus starting a new practice, versus starting a new sponsored practice. With the advent of new Federal fraud and abuse regulations, hospitals may no longer have wide flexibility in sponsoring new medical practices.

The advantages and disadvantages of solo practice are discussed in Table 1.2. The general advantages and disadvantages of being in a group practice (in addition to the converse of those listed under solo practice) are listed in Table 1.3.

As a new career physician, the time pressures of solo practice can be so demanding that it may be extremely disruptive of family life. For example, receiving telephone calls from patients night after night may result in unhealthy sleep deprivation for you and your spouse. In addition, starting a solo practice in terms of mastering all of the complicated financial and paperwork requirements necessary may detract significantly from time available for patient care. By joining an established group practice immediately after residency, learning and mastering the paperwork and political aspects of medical practice will be easier. If group practice becomes a less than ideal situation, you can then take the knowledge gained initially and apply it to your own solo practice.

There are three options for entering into solo practice:

1. Buy an existing practice
2. Start a new practice
3. Start a new sponsored practice

Table 1.4 lists the general advantages and disadvantages of buying an existing practice, whereas those of starting a new practice, in addition to those previously mentioned, are included in Table 1.5.

Table 1.1
Career Options After Residency

- Private practice
  - Solo practice
    - Buy an existing practice
    - Start a new practice
    - Start a sponsored practice
  - Join a practice
  - (one or more partners)
  - Join a group medical practice
  - Join a clinic
  - (multispecialty)
  - Work for a health maintenance organization (HMO)
  - Work as a hospital based physician
  - Be a free-standing facility physician
  - Be employed by a nonhospital company
  - Be employed by a pharmaceutical company
- "Pure" academic
  - Clinical
  - Research
  - Clinical and Research
  - Administrative
  - Teaching
- Mixed academic-private practice
  - University hospital teaching service
  - Private hospital teaching service
- Government employment
  - Public Health Service
  - Indian Health Service
  - Foreign services
  - Various agencies (Centers for Disease Control, Food and Drug Administration, etc.)
- Military
  - Commission/active duty
  - Reserves/National Guard
- "Migratory"
  - Locum tenens
  - Cruise ships
  - Overseas companies
  - Peace Corps
  - Church Missionary services
- Do another residency or fellowship
- Take a year off and do something else

Table 1.2
Solo Practice

Advantages	Disadvantages
Control over both financial decisions and decisions about patient medical care	No time off (if maintaining 24-hour availability to patients and consultants)
Control over office structure, staff selection, and staff procedures	No generated income if not actively working for a period of time (i.e., vacations or illness)
Control over own work schedule	Less access or ease of consultation or advice
Greater freedom and independence to change the practice as necessary	No ready-made buyer for the practice if you decide to sell (as would exist if you had a partner)
Not undertaking responsibility for the actions of other physicians	The tendency to feel somewhat lonely or overwhelmed without having another physician with whom to share the workload

Hospitals or communities may help defray the start-up costs of a new practice seen as contributing to their overall mission or welfare. This can take several forms. The hospital or community may provide office space or a clinic facility, or they may provide money or loans directly for practice start-up costs. In other instances, they may provide some support personnel or computer equipment to take care of some of the business aspects of the practice. Make certain, though, that there are no disagreeable strings attached to the sponsorship arrangement, e.g., the sponsoring hospital insists that all patient referrals for admission be to that particular hospital. If it is the only hospital you are going to utilize anyway, then, of course, this is no problem. However, if there is a choice of several local hospitals, this covenant may be too restrictive for your practice. Also, it should be clear whether the sponsorship money is being donated or will need to be repaid and at what rate. The use of "sponsorship practice" had been increasing by both hospitals and communities that were recruiting physicians, especially primary care physicians. However, recent

Table 1.3
Group Practice

Advantages	Disadvantages
More ability to diversify or subspecialize and develop expertise in a particular area	A general loss of independence
Ability to schedule important family events for days when not on-call	The need to discuss and compromise before making any decision about the operation of the practice
The patient "will not feel left out in the cold" if you leave the practice, because other members can provide continued care	If entering as a junior member of the practice, you may find yourself on the "short end" of on-call scheduling and of the relative pay scale
Ease in keeping up with new medical developments by having easier access to consultation with your partner	Having to accept procedural aspects of the office and the existing office staff, whether you agree or not
More readily obtainable social activities for your family with the families of your partner physicians	The specific medical practice techniques of other member(s) of the group may be old-fashioned or objectionable

Federal legislation restricting the ability of physicians to refer patients to facilities in which the physicians have a financial interest has made "sponsored practice" more difficult. You should review the specifics of any such arrangement with a lawyer to make certain that the Federal guidelines are not violated.

Joining a multispecialty clinic is another option within private practice (Table 1.6). These clinics may vary in size from a few to over 100 physicians. Joining a health maintenance organization (HMO) is becoming a more common career choice for graduating resident physicians as these organizations expand (Table 1.7).

The next type of private practice option to consider is that of a hospital-based physician. Radiologists, pathologists, anesthesiologists and emergency physicians are the major groups that fall into this category. In cases where these physician positions are structured as groups contracting with the hospital or facility, all of the above considerations about group practices apply. However,

Table 1.4
Buying a Practice

Advantages	Disadvantages
The physical structure, office staff, paperwork, and computer systems are already established	The practice may have procedures and/or physical facilities that are not ideal
Established patients will provide a reliable source of income from the outset	The initial fee to purchase the practice may be between $50,000 and $500,000
Availability of consulting physicians is already developed	There may be some office staff whom you find unacceptable
Ready access to medical records of patients' prior medical care within the practice	The patients of the practice may decide to go to another established physician of whom they have prior knowledge
Time to concentrate on patient care initially because do not have to spend time interviewing potential employees for hire	The physician selling the practice may have a poor relationship with other consultant physicians and/or hospitals, which may be applied to you at the beginning of practice
An established, experienced office staff can provide advice on avoiding "political" mistakes early in practice	The physician selling the practice may return in the future and "steal" patients back from the practice

Table 1.5
New Practice

Advantages	Disadvantages
Freedom and independence in terms of physical structure and scheduling	Uncertain income until a patient base is established
Start-up costs are more directly retrievable than when purchasing another practice	Greater initial time commitment involved in hiring new office staff
More control over the patients seen in the practice	Greater initial time commitment in having to write the policy manuals for the practice

Table 1.6
Multispecialty Clinic Practice

Advantages	Disadvantages
Initial income is usually good in that many clinics pay their physicians on a salary basis; even if you are a separate practitioner in terms of income, the clinic essentially guarantees you referral of a steady supply of patients	Income may be less than in a single specialty practice or in a solo practice
The opportunity exists to interact with a number different physicians, making consultation very easy to obtain	Clinical overhead financial charges may be greater for certain specialties
A clinic's physical structure and equipment tend to be more complete, and more support services can generally be offered than in a single specialty	There may be some disagreeable administrative or paperwork requirements by the clinic
Generally, only patients with some demonstrated form of adequate health insurance coverage are accepted, making patient payment fairly reliable	There may be a requirement to refer patients for a particular consultation to other physicians within the clinic as opposed to an outside physician

where these physician arrangements are run more like an HMO or group multispecialty clinic, the advantages and disadvantages of these types of practice listed above should be considered.

Working for a free-standing facility, such as an "urgent care" center or "minor emergencies" center is another career option to consider (Table 1.8). There are thousands of these facilities across the country. Some are run like small hospital emergency departments whereas others are run more like private practice offices.

Additional options for careers in private practice include working for a private company or factory as the "company physician" (Table 1.9) or as an "occupational health physician." Most medium-sized companies, in fact, do not require a full-time physician but utilize someone already in an office or hospital-

Table 1.7
HMO Practice

Advantages	Disadvantages
Generally limited work hours and on-call responsibilities compared with other forms of private practice	The administrative rules and requirements of the HMO may prohibit physicians from practicing what is considered to be in the patient's best interest (restrictions on ordering certain tests, seeing the patient at certain intervals, etc., which may not be directly related to patient care considerations)
Guaranteed salaried income	The income may be significantly lower than in other private practice arrangements
A "guaranteed" supply of patients	Income may be tied to utilization factors such that it will drop with increased patient utilization of health care services within the HMO
Perhaps less paperwork in general related to billing compared with other forms of practice	Possible restrictions on choice of facilities in which the patients can be treated
Preventive medicine may be more appropriately emphasized and supported	Patients may be unhappy with the various restrictions of the HMO care plan

based practice on a part-time basis to satisfy their employee health care needs. Generally, only the larger companies with at least several hundred employees need to have a full-time company-based physician. Many of the disadvantages listed above for an HMO physician apply as well to a company physician. In addition, there may be an almost "adversarial" relationship with either patients and/or management. This occurs when the patient's perception of injury or illness conflicts with the company's interest in having the employee return to work and the physician is pressured from both sides.

One final option to consider in private practice is a position with one of the pharmaceutical companies. Generally, the pharmaceutical companies are seeking physicians with research back-

Table 1.8
Free-standing Facility Practice

Advantages	Disadvantages
Set hours, predictable schedule, usually no "late night" work time	The equipment, lab capability, and x-ray capability in the facility may be limited compared to that of a private practice clinic or hospital
No on-call responsibilities	There may not be a direct relationship between the facility and a hospital or primary and specialty practices, which might then impede patient referral
May be better equipped than a private office	The overhead costs at this type of facility often exceed that of a private office facility
Salaried; guaranteed income independent of patient volume	The patient population utilizing a free-standing facility may be less reliable or return for repeat visits less regularly than in an established office-based practice
Can take vacation	Lack of established rapport and follow-up
Can serve as "transition" job	May directly compete with established office practices

grounds who are interested in pharmaceutical research and promotion of use of pharmaceuticals. Their need for physicians directly out of residency is very limited and the number of positions that open up at any one time is also limited. However, this is an option to consider if you enjoy research and administrative work. The patient care aspects for most physicians working for pharmaceutical companies are very limited. The initial income is often significantly less than in private practice. However, most senior level physicians employed by pharmaceutical companies have incomes above the median for physicians in private practice. Obviously, on-call responsibilities and night work responsibilities with a pharmaceutical company would generally be either nonexistent or very limited.

Table 1.9
Company Physician Practice

Advantages	Disadvantages
Work hours are generally limited and on-call responsibilities usually nonexistent	Often there may not be a formal arrangement with other health care facilities or other physicians leading to a feeling of isolation
The supply of patients is obviously "guaranteed" by the company itself	Company policies may conflict with health care measures applicable to certain health problems

"PURE ACADEMIC" PRACTICE

In deciding on a career in academic medicine versus private practice, it is very important to assess your own personality traits and temperament. To succeed in academic practice, an interest in teaching as well as an aptitude for lecturing and manuscript preparation are important. Patience and flexibility are essential in guiding the physicians in training under you while still allowing them to develop their own practice style. In surgical specialties, this necessitates increasingly turning over the surgical management or performance of cases to residents as they mature. Strictly "hands-on" physicians not comfortable delegating significant aspects of patient care to someone with lesser training probably should not go into an academic environment.

To those who enjoy an academic career, the rewards of teaching and interacting with physicians in training make up for the usually lower salaries found in academia. However, the payment gap between academics and private practice has narrowed in recent years and there is considerable overlap in practice income. Academics, in addition to clinical work, has the added responsibilities and time commitments of lecturing and research. The political and administrative requirements of an academic career are somewhat different and usually greater than in private practice.

The four aspects of careers within academics are:

1. Clinical practice
2. Research
3. Administration
4. Teaching

Most academic faculty are expected to perform some combination of the four, with the relative contribution of each aspect (it is hoped) tailored to the individual's interests and aptitudes. Recently, greater emphasis has been placed on patient care and its generation of revenue to support the academic institution, leading to opportunities within academic settings that are essentially 100% clinically oriented. This type of position may not require research or didactic teaching outside of the clinical setting and may combine rewarding aspects of academic practice with higher financial reward. However, advancement in most academic medical institutions requires adherence to the old dictum of "publish or perish." The new junior faculty member interested in an academic career can relatively easily initiate some clinical and chart review projects that do not require obtaining grants or significant funding. Opportunities to socialize with peers are often enhanced in the academic setting as compared with private practice.

MIXED ACADEMIC AND PRIVATE PRACTICE

This type of career option combines a lot of the nicest aspects of academic practice with those of private practice. These types of positions are available at some university hospital teaching services and at a number of private hospitals that are affiliated with residency programs. In these types of positions your main clinical responsibilities involve direct patient care, but residents would rotate through your service under your supervision. Responsibilities for teaching these residents usually center just around clinical supervision. In general, these types of positions pay as well as anything else in private practice and yet you still get some teaching contact with residents. In addition, the "hassle" factors of academic practice are usually not present, namely the pressure to do research or conduct teaching outside the clinical arena.

GOVERNMENT

Government positions for physicians exist within the Public Health Service and its subagency, the Indian Health Service. Recipients of National Health Program scholarships for medical school have practice commitments postresidency with this agency, although others may opt to start their career in such service. The pay in these agencies tends to be lower than that in private practice. Government positions are also available with the

Centers for Disease Control, headquartered in Atlanta, the Food and Drug Administration, headquartered in Washington, DC, as well as other government agencies. These include the U.S. Foreign Service, providing physician service to U.S. embassies and other U.S. national facilities abroad, and the Veterans Administration. Significant consideration is given to experience and prior government service in filling these positions, making it somewhat difficult for recent residency graduates to obtain such employment. Security clearance procedures for Foreign Service positions also require a long time period before employment.

MILITARY

Physicians in the military are commissioned as officers in the Medical Corps. The amount of paperwork in military practice is probably less than in the typical civilian private practice. Military pay scales tend to be significantly lower than private practice but have been improving in recent years. When the military benefits of housing allowance, PX privileges, malpractice insurance coverage, Continuing Medical Education (CME) time and funding, access to military travel systems, clerical support staff, and facilities are taken into consideration, the compensation in military practice can approach that in civilian practice.

Physicians may apply for a commission and active duty or may join the National Guard or Reserves. Active duty service entails a full-time position and commitment, usually of 4 years with an additional required follow-on time of 4 or more years in the Reserves. Obtaining a commission with the necessary background checks requires several months, so if you are considering a military position, this process should be started early.

The military Reserves and National Guard fund a number of full-time physician positions to staff various readiness and administrative units; however, most of their physician opportunities are part-time positions. The rules for participation and the actual time commitments are much more lax for physicians than they are for other Reserve or Guard personnel. Generally, the time commitment would be one weekend (often just 9:00 to 5:00 each day and not necessarily the whole weekend), or even less a month, as well as a 2-week summer camp. For physicians, this summer camp experience often involves working at a large military medical facility or traveling with a military unit for field exercises overseas. The pay scale in the Reserves and National Guard is not high but makes for a nice reliable extra source of income. The only real drawback to Reserve and National Guard commitment is, of course, the possibility of call-up to active duty. Being called to active duty has much more serious effects on a solo or small group practice than on a large group, multispecialty clinic, or academic-based practice.

MIGRATORY

The "migratory" category includes locum tenens work, work as a cruise ship doctor, work with overseas companies, and work with the Peace Corps or church missionary services. These are viable options if you are unsure of your long-term goals or have a hiatus in your career.

There are a number of organizations that serve as clearing houses for locum tenens positions, and such work can be easily arranged through these companies. A locum tenens position involves operating a physician's practice for a period of time, ranging from 2 weeks to a year, after which time the practice is returned to the original physician. A number of physicians in private practice may opt for coverage from a locum tenens physician intermittently to allow an extended vacation or because of temporary health problems. The advantages of locum tenens positions include the ability to experience different practice styles and settings. In addition, the salary in a locum tenens position is generally guaranteed. Locum tenens positions also exist in Emergency Departments and clinics and allow a greater flexibility for the nomadic soul or the physician as yet unsure of long-term goals or where to settle. See Appendix 1.1 for addresses of some locum tenens firms.

Cruise ship lines recruit physicians to staff their ships' medical facilities for vacation cruises. The workload in these positions is generally light, although the physician usually is on-call 24 hours per day and may not be allowed much shore leave during the cruise. The pay and related perks are usually generous. When considering such positions, it is important to make sure that the cruise ship has adequate equipment, pharmaceutical inventory, support staff, and access to emergency transportation should an illness or injury aboard ship exceed the ship's capabilities.

For those interested in practicing medicine in foreign countries, options include working for a U.S. company with overseas work commitments, working for the Peace Corps, or working with a church missionary service. Overseas jobs with private business firms tend to pay very well with additional benefits, but are often restrictive in terms of practice style. Also, these positions may only be operable for limited periods of time. Contracts with this type of company should be carefully scrutinized. Significant personal U.S. income tax reduction may be available for such out of country employment. However, some countries restrict sending money out of the country, requiring you to spend your entire salary there. If high income is not a consideration, the Peace Corps or church missionary service options are worthwhile, and the human service rewards can be great.

OTHER OPTIONS

Doing another residency or fellowship becomes an important option for those unhappy with their specialty choice in medicine. Doing another residency would usually involve starting over in a new residency program but some advanced standing is sometimes granted. Undertaking a fellowship is another option, allowing for subspecialization. The length of most fellowships is almost the same as residency programs (2–3 years). Fellowship salaries tend to be $5000–6000 a year higher than those of residents. Though starting a new residency or fellowship can be strenuous and difficult, it may be preferable to continuing in a specialty career that is uninteresting or unrewarding.

Some resident physicians may chose to take a year off and do something else (study music, play professional sports, etc.). With sufficient financial means this may be a viable option. An extended "vacation" of this type, however, may be viewed unfavorably by prospective physician employers in the future. When a protracted time period away from medical practice occurs, the "use it or lose it" factor becomes important, making return to practice increasingly difficult.

An additional option to mention is the least desirable one—changing careers completely. This means you would be discarding your 7–8 years of investment in medical training to undertake a completely unrelated career. Once committed to another career, it would be very difficult to restart back in medicine. You should probably undertake this option only if you have a truly wonderful "once in a lifetime" opportunity (such as a major business take-over). Even in this situation the best option would be to maintain at least part-time involvement in medicine in addition to the major career switch.

HOW TO FIND PRIVATE PRACTICE POSITIONS

For those interested in entering private practice, it is appropriate to start investigating practice opportunities early in the last year of residency. The advertisement section at the back of each of the specialty medical journals are readily available sources of practice opportunities. Some advertisements will be by so-called "head hunter" groups or "search consultants" who are retained to recruit candidates for medical practices. These recruiters rarely charge a fee to the applicant but rather receive a "finders fee" from the client who has retained them to fill the position. When dealing with such a recruiter, it is important for you to clearly specify all your interests and requirements so that your time is not wasted investigating or considering positions that would not be of interest to you. In the past, such physician recruiters were often retained to fill only the difficult, less than desirable positions; however, that is no longer true, and a large number of very desirable positions are marketed through physician recruiters. Beware that if you exclusively use a recruitment firm (with its attendant placement fees) this may make you a less desirable candidate with some potential employers (because of the direct cost to them).

Another major source of potential leads in seeking practice opportunities includes state or national medical business or specialty scientific meetings. Booths and/or seminars are presented at most of these meetings to disseminate information about practice opportunities. Another productive source of potential opportunities includes the state and county medical associations in the locations in which you are interested, which may be contacted by mail with requests for information on any practice opportunities in their geographic areas. If searching for opportunities in a limited geographic area, the hospital's Chief of Staff or human resources office may be contacted by phone or mail requesting similar information.

Although more expensive, personal advertisement (of your availability and interests) in the specialty journals, specifying interest in practice positions or openings may prove worthwhile.

The text should include the best way for you to be contacted (phone or address for correspondence). In general, this type of advertising as a resident is not necessary because the recruiting networks are so extensive and interlocking that there should be plenty of practice opportunities to evaluate with only minimal effort. There are two national registries listed in the Appendix 1.1 that will publish a brief version of your curriculum vitae, practice and geographic preferences, and availability dates. Although easy to access, most people in the recruiting business do not seem to utilize these two registries frequently.

To summarize then, a good way to start looking for practice opportunities involves following this sequence:

1. Determine your career goals and the type of practice you want.
2. Scan your specialty journal job advertisements and make direct phone contacts of interesting-sounding positions.
3. Contact one or more recruitment firms to let them know you are interested in looking at positions.
4. Attend your medical specialty regional or national meetings and directly follow-up any interesting advertised positions.
5. Contact the AMA placement office if you are an AMA member.

See the first part of Chapter 5 for a more detailed sequence of recommended actions in looking for practice opportunities.

Appendix 1.1

Medical Jobs—Contact Phone Numbers and Addresses

NATIONAL CV REGISTRIES

AMA Physician Placement Register
515 North State Street
Chicago, IL 60610
213–464–5000
(published bimonthly)

National Physicians Register
8 Park Place
Boston, MA 02116
800–342–1007
(published 6 times annually)

LOCUM TENENS GROUPS

Locum Tenens Service
Physicians Career Resource
American Medical Association
P.O Box 10012
Chicago, IL 60610
1–800–955–3565

Locum Tenens, Inc.
A Division of Jackson and Coker
115 Perimeter Center Place
Suite 380—JDLT1
—AEML1
Atlanta, GA 30346
1–800–272–2707 extension 56
extension 62

MedStaff
National Staffing, Inc.
1–800–476–7566

Cheree Richards
EMSA Limited Partnership
100 NW 70th Avenue
Ft. Lauderdale, FL 33317
1–800–443–3672

Physician International
Locum Tenens Division
4-ER Vermont Street
Buffalo, NY 15213
1–800–622–4062

Comp Health
1–800–453–3030
(Salt Lake City, UT; Atlanta, GA)

IPR Medical, Inc.
7207 West Greenfield Avenue
Milwaukee, WI 53214
1–800–966–3627

Locum Medical Group
30100 Chagrin Boulevard
Cleveland, OH 44124
1–800–752–5515

Medical Doctor Associates, Inc.
3495 Holcomb Bridge Road
Norcross, GA 30092
1–800–780–3500 extension 348

KRON Medical Corporation
725 Airport Road, 3rd Floor
Chapel Hill, NC 27514
1–800–MEDICAL

Vista Staffing Solutions
675 E 2100 South, Suite 390
Salt Lake City, UT 84106
1–800–366–1884

FOREIGN MEDICAL POSITIONS
LIST OF CONTACTS

American Medical Association
Physicians' International Placement Services
515 North State Street
Chicago, IL 60610
1–800–AMA–3211 (for AMA members)

National Council for International Health
1701 K Street NW
Suite 600
Washington, DC 20006
202–833–5900

Project Concern International
3550 Afton Road
San Diego, CA 92123
619–279–9690

International Medical Corps
5933 W. Century Boulevard
Suite 310
Los Angeles, CA 90045
310–670–0800

International Resume Committee
386 Park Avenue South
New York, NY 10016
212–679–0010

World Health Organization
P.O. Box 5284
Church Street Station
New York, NY 10249

World Health Organization
Fellowship Selection Committee
Health Resources and Services Administration
5600 Fishers Lane, Room 14–14
Rockville, MD 20857
301–443–6152

American Medical International, Inc.
International Recruiter
9465 Wilshire Boulevard, Suite 307
Beverly Hills, CA 90212
213–858–1125

Hospital Corporation of America International
P.O. Box 550
Nashville, TN 37202
615–327–9551

Executive Health Search Consultants, Inc.
400 Plaza Drive
Harmon Meadow
Secaucus, NJ 07094
1–800–223–8978

Department of Commerce
Office of the Near East
Room H–2039
U.S. Department of Commerce
Washington, DC 20239
202–377–5767

Public Health Service
Bureau of Health Manpower
Center Building
3700 East–West Highway
Hyattsville, MD 20782

Indian Health Service Recruitment Program
Twinbrook Metro Plaza Building
Suite 100
12300 Twinbrook Parkway
Rockville, MD 20852
1–800–962–2817
In Maryland 301–443–4242

PHARMACEUTICAL COMPANY POSITIONS

Sampson, Neill, & Wilkins, Inc.
543 Valley Road
Upper Montclair, NJ 07043
201–783–9600
1–800–634–0837

MILITARY MEDICAL RECRUITING

Air National Guard
301–981–8407 (collect)

Air Force Opportunity Center
P.O. Box 3506
Capitol Heights, MD 20791–3506
1–800–423–USAF

USAF Recruiting Service / RSH
Randolpoh AFB, TX 78150–5421

Navy
1–800–327–NAVY

Army Opportunities
Army Medical Corps
P.O. Box 7700
Clifton, NJ 07015–9865
1–800–USA ARMY

MISSIONARY/VOLUNTEER CONTACTS

Peace Corps
Volunteer Partners Program
9th Floor, 1990 K Street, NW
Washington, DC 20526
1–800–424–8580 extension 2238

Lutheran World Relief
212–532–6350

Mexican Mission Ministries, Inc.
517–787–3543

Mennonite Board of Missionaries
219–294–7523

Missionaries of Africa
201–561–3077

Overseas Missions Department
Evangelical Free Church of America
612–866–3343

Project Hope
Project Hope Health Sciences Education Center
Millwood, VA 22646
703–837–2100

World Gospel Mission
P.O. Box 948
Marion, IN 46952–0948
317–664–7331

World Medical Mission, Inc.
P.O. Box 3000
Boone, NC 28607
704–262–1980

A reference list for physician service opportunities abroad was published in **JAMA** 1993;270(5):567–571; 89 organizations (with contact phone numbers and addresses) are listed in this reference.

Chapter 2

Choosing the Community in Which to Settle

GOAL

The goal of this chapter is to present the range of items to consider in selecting a community in which to start medical practice.

MAJOR CONSIDERATIONS

Major items you should consider when choosing where to settle after residency include the region of the country, the type of topography, the climate, and the population size of the community itself.

There is a great deal of variability as to what constitute regional boundaries within this country. Some sample groupings of states within regions are shown in Table 2.1. In selecting an area in which to live and work, modify the groupings of states according to your knowledge, experience, and preference.

Within any region, there is, of course, variation in topography. The area's topography can be important aesthetically as well as in relation to the types of outdoor recreation available. Topographical classifications to consider include mountains, flatlands, coastal, nearby rivers/lakes, desert, and piedmont or "rolling" hills.

Community size can be classified simply:

< 20,000 people—town
20,000–40,000 people—small city
40,000–60,000 people—medium city
60,000–100,000 people—medium/large city
> 100,000 people—large city
> 500,000 people—very large city

Table 2.1
Regions in the United States

Northeast	Southeast	Midwest	Northwest	Far West	Southwest	Plains	Desert
Maine	Maryland	Minnesota	Idaho	Montana	Utah	Indiana	Idaho
Vermont	Virginia	Wisconsin	Washington	Idaho	Colorado	Illinois	Utah
New Hampshire	Delaware	Michigan	Oregon	Wyoming	Arizona	Missouri	Nevada
Massachusetts	North Carolina	Iowa		Utah	New Mexico	Iowa	Arizona
Connecticut	South Carolina	Illinois		Nevada	Nevada	Texas	New Mexico
Rhode Island	Georgia	Indiana		New Mexico		Oklahoma	Wyoming
New York	Florida	Ohio		Arizona		Kansas	Colorado
New Jersey	Alabama	Missouri		Colorado		Nebraska	California
Pennsylvania	Tennessee					Texas	
	Mississippi					South Dakota	
	Louisiana					Montana	
						North Dakota	

Mountains	Cold Winter	East Coast	Pacific Coast	Gulf Coast	Appalachia	South
Maine	Maine	Maine	Washington	Florida	Georgia	Maryland
New Hampshire	Vermont	New Hampshire	Oregon	Alabama	North Carolina	Virginia
Vermont	New Hampshire	Massachusetts	California	Mississippi	Tennessee	West Virginia
New York	New York	Connecticut		Louisiana	Kentucky	North Carolina
Pennsylvania	Wisconsin	Rhode Island		Texas	Virginia	South Carolina
West Virginia	Michigan	New York			West Virginia	Tennessee
Virginia	Minnesota	New Jersey				Kentucky
North Carolina	North Dakota	Maryland				Georgia
Tennessee	South Dakota	Delaware				Alabama
Kentucky	Montana	Virginia				Mississippi
Montana	Idaho	North Carolina				Louisiana
Wyoming	Utah	South Carolina				Texas
Colorado	Wyoming	Georgia				Arkansas
Utah		Florida				Florida
New Mexico						
Arizona						
Nevada						
Idaho						
Washington						
Oregon						
California						

The size of the community may be a more important factor than region, climate, or topography in determining you and your spouse's happiness with location and lifestyle. Obviously, smaller towns and cities generally have fewer social and cultural activities than larger cities but have fewer transportation difficulties and, perhaps, less crime.

In addition to such personal considerations regarding the selection of a community in which to settle, there are professional concerns about medical practice within the community that need to be examined. Will established practitioners welcome you as a new physician in the community? If you are actively recruited by the physicians in the community, your presence is obviously desired and referrals should be forthcoming. However, if you are moving unsolicited into a community, you may be viewed as "unwanted competition." It would also be wise for you to investigate the degree of competition among medical facilities in the community, as well as among different existing groups of physicians. Where stiff competition already exists or there exists an apparent local physician surplus, it may be very difficult to start a practice and, consequently, your initial financial returns may be low.

The local availability and quality of pharmacy and support services (such as radiology and medical laboratory) at the hospitals or medical facilities should also be investigated. Whether the area participates in any regional medical referral system, such as a formal trauma system or referral of high-risk obstetrics, neonates, and others to specialty centers is important to determine if your practice would rely on seeing such cases. It should also be determined how the local emergency medical services or prehospital care system might influence your practice.

Carefully evaluate the size and capabilities of the hospitals at which you would be seeking admission privileges. Obviously, smaller community hospitals with limited ICU facilities cannot well support physicians whose main area of practice involves specialized intensive care. Opportunities in cardiology, for example, might also be limited if the hospital does not possess cardiovascular surgery potential. The financial stability and long-range plans of the local hospital are of concern. There have been quite a number of hospital closures across the country in the last decade, many of which were in rural areas or small towns. For practices in which in-hospital care constitutes an important component, closing or downgrading of the only local hospital could be devastating to your practice. If there is more than one hospital in the immediate area, maintaining admitting privileges at more than one would be a "safer" situation.

OTHER FACTORS TO CONSIDER

1. *The general economy and economic stability of the community.* You should try to determine whether the community is on an economic upswing or downswing. If the community is dependent upon a single industry or single military base for much of its revenue, obviously it could have severe economic problems that would reflect on your practice if the industry or base suddenly closed. Having a diversified economic base in a community tends to make it much more stable economically.
2. *The local government and whether it is supportive of the medical facilities and physicians in the community.* To assess this, you should determine if local government officials are on the board of directors of the hospital, and if there are any major political problems between the local government and the hospital or medical practices. You should also find out the state and local tax structure, and what community services are supported by taxes.
3. *Zoning considerations regarding the site of your office or clinic.* If you are planning to build a new office or clinic, it is important to make sure that the local zoning would allow such construction. In addition, if joining another physician's practice, it is important to determine that the zoning laws do not prohibit practice in the existent clinic or location (if the physician operates an office out of his or her home, zoning laws may not allow a second, unrelated person to work there full-time).
4. *Crime rate.* This is an important consideration, especially for those with a spouse or family. As part of this assessment, you may want to determine the location and availability of local police units.
5. *Housing.* You should assess the general availability of housing, and the cost range. If you are planning to build a new home, assess the availability and cost for undeveloped lots in the area. Determine whether the type of home you want (condominium, townhouse, residential neighborhood, farm) is

available within reasonable commuting distance to the hospital or office. You may have to determine whether greater daily commuting distance or greater property value is more important to you.

6. *Local schools.* You should assess the facilities and equipment of the local schools, the average test performance of the students on national standardized examinations, and the relative distance from your planned residence of the school. If your children have any particular aptitudes or interests, you should determine if the local schools have programs specific for these aptitudes or interests. If you find the public schools in the area are lacking, look into the availability and cost of local private schools.
7. *Stores/shopping.* In smaller communities the availability of stores and other retail businesses may be very limited. The need to drive a considerable distance to shop may constitute a significant drawback for the community.
8. *Recreational opportunities and facilities.* This includes the availability of various forms of outdoor recreation as well as the availability of local movies, concerts, and theaters, and other social activities.
9. *The local highway system and general transportation accessibility.* If you need or like to travel frequently, locating near major highways and/or an airport may be important.
10. *Distance from family or friends.* This is often the overriding concern in choosing a particular community. Staying in geographic proximity to your close relatives can certainly ease the difficulty of arranging frequent babysitting for your children.
11. *Presence of religious congregations of your faith or denomination.*
12. *Ethnic considerations.* If you have social practices, religious beliefs, or even a regional accent markedly at variance with those in the community, you may have a hard time "fitting in," which may translate into lack of patient referrals.
13. *Spouse happiness.* The wishes and long-term goals of your spouse or significant other should obviously be considered and their input sought from the outset. Even though listed last, this is probably the most important consideration. The spouse or significant other may need to explore employment opportunities available in his or her chosen field.

Writing down a list of the particular factors that are considered desirable in a community with your spouse doing likewise is a good way to start in selecting a community in which to settle. You should establish a rank order of relative importance for each item on the list. Your list can then be compared with your spouse's, and determination can be made as to which factors are imperative and which are negotiable.

Prior to visiting a community, a number of matters should be researched. Generally, most hospitals and larger group practices will supply you with preprinted data about the community and region. If not, this information can usually be obtained from the local Chamber of Commerce or the state Bureau of Tourism. Reviewing this information before making a trip will help focus on what facts you need to obtain on the trip itself. Review of the listings in the local telephone directory (Yellow Pages) allows assessment of physicians and their specialties, clinic arrangements, locations of their offices, and organization into groups. The Yellow Pages, in fact, are probably a more reliable listing of local physicians than can be obtained even from the county medical society. Often, a number of physicians practicing locally will not be members of the local or state medical society, but almost all physicians in private practice will have a phone listing.

It is never advisable to take a position in a community without having actually visited the community. Your overall impression of the community can change greatly from a visit compared with your anticipated impressions from written information alone. Making a trip to a community without making specific appointments with anyone is appropriate if you are unsure about the opportunities. However, if you are seriously considering a position in a given community, it is wise to set up a number of interviews. Consider talking with a bank manager, a real estate officer, a school principal, a pharmacist, and a religious leader. You should formally interview with a representative of the hospital administration, other physicians in the group, potential referral physicians, and one or more of the administrative nurses at the hospital or clinic. While in the community, you can pick up a local paper and a local real estate listing for more information on the community itself. If the community is in a region with which you are unfamiliar, consider making more than one trip there at different seasons of the year to make certain that the locale still seems agreeable regardless of the season of the year.

Before spending any money to visit a community for a possible position, determine if travel costs will be reimbursed by the hospital, the recruiting physician group, or the "headhunter agency" that is marketing the position. Very often most of the travel costs for at least one interview trip will be borne by the recruiting party. Most of them also recognize the importance of a spouse's input and will also pay for at least one trip to the community by your spouse. If making a trip into a community by aircraft or train, obtain a car either by loan or rental to drive around the community. This will provide a better feel for the community than just being shuttled between the airport and the hospital or clinic as part of the interview trip.

A very useful initial source to plan a "community education trip" is the American Automobile Association (AAA). Members can obtain excellent maps and tourist brochures of any area in the country, and the staff can advise travel routes. AAA membership is very inexpensive and well worth the travel assistance and discounts it provides.

Chapter 3

Preparing Curriculum Vitae and the Interview Process

GOALS

The goals of this chapter are to present a method to write a complete curriculum vitae, to provide guidelines for conducting oneself at a job interview, and to provide a checklist of the most important information to obtain from a job interview.

INTRODUCTION

Careful preparation of a written curriculum vitae (CV) is one of the most important steps in preparing for medical practice. Review of applicants' CVs by the employer is the first and most important step in choosing good candidates for a position. This is common to almost all physician positions, and because attractive positions have a relatively large number of applicants, poorly prepared or incomplete CVs are generally excluded from further consideration as part of the initial screening. While you are a resident, take the time to prepare and complete a well-worded CV. This will be well worthwhile when you reach the point of making formal job applications. The following is a list of "nevers" regarding CV writing and submission:

1. Never submit handwritten CVs.
2. Never have the CV printed on nonstandard size (other than 8 1/2 by 11 inch) paper.
3. Never use such things as copied pages from medical specialist directories, telephone book listings, or staff brochure listings.
4. Never submit a CV without a formal "cover letter".

Table 3.1
Sample Curriculum Vitae

I. *Personal Data*

Name: (complete name)
Date of Birth: (month/day/year)
Place of Birth: (town, state, ± country)
Citizenship: (U.S.A. or other)
*Social Security Number:
Spouse: (full name)
Spouse's occupation:
Children: (names and year of birth, i.e., "Mark Spencer, born 1980")
*Hobbies: (list 2 to 6)
Language Fluency: (English, ± any others)
Home Address: (current complete address)
Home Telephone:
Office Address:
Office Telephone:
FAX:
*Best time to receive calls (list hours and where to call)
*Denote address/phone number at which you prefer to receive correspondence.

II. *Education*

High School	(name)
	(town, state)
	Attendance (years)
College	(name)
	(town, state)
	Attendance (years)

	Degree(s) (type, subject)
	Awards or Offices held (list)
Medical School	(name)
	(city, state)
	Attendance (years)
	Degree (M.D., D.O.)
	Awards (list)
	References upon request
Internship	(type)
	(department)
	(medical center or institution name)
	(city, state)
	Dates (19__ to 19__)
Residency	(type)
	(department)
	(medical center or institution name)
	(city, state)
	(Dates 19__ to 19__)
Fellowship	(type)
	(department)
	(medical center or institution name)
	(city, state)
	Dates (19__ to 19__)

III. *Preresidency Professional Experience*

Ward orderly (etc.), hospital name, city, state, month/year of service

Next position (type), hospital or organization name, city, state month/year of service or work (list each separate position)

Military service (could be listed as a separate section; include rank attained and locations of major periods of service)

Table 3.1 (continued)
Sample Curriculum Vitae

IV. *Medical Practice Experience*
- Your title or position, hospital or practice name, city, state, dates
- *Reference person name (list a separate reference person for each position held)
- Title, clinic name, city, state, dates (denote "moonlighting" or "weekends")
- List each separate position held (proceed from earliest to most recent in order)

V. *Current Professional Activities*
- Membership in societies and organizations
  - (American Medical Association, years)
  - (Specialty association, years)
  - (Honorary Society, years)
- Committees and appointments
  - (Hospital committee name, hospital name, years)
  - (Regional committee name, organization, years)
  - (*Major* community service organization, years)
- *Recent selected CME activities ("further list of conferences attended available on request")
  (list 5 or 6, of the most recently attended (*not* more) including title, city in which held, dates)

VI. *Medical Licensure*
- State(s) medical license, number, dates (when license active)
- *Federal DEA number, dates (for security you may want to just list that you have a DEA number but state it is "available on request")
- Other specialty licenses

VII. *Certifications*
- Board Certification
  - Name of board, type of exam, dates, note if passed
  - *Scores

Fellow of ____ College, dates
Board Recertifications
Other Certifications
ACLS (provider or instructor), city, state, dates
ATLS (provider or instructor), city, state, dates
PALS or APLS
Diplomate of National Board of Medical Examiners (number, data passed)

VIII. *Publications*

Journal Articles
Authors: Title. Journal and Year; Volume (issue):
Page numbers.

Abstracts
Authors: Title. Journal and Year; Volume (issue):
Page numbers.

Books and book chapters
For book chapters
Authors: Title, in Editor's name (ed.): Title of book, ed number. City, State, Publisher, Year, Volume if any, Page numbers.
For book
Author(s): Title of book ed number. City, State, Publisher, Year.

IX. *Presentations*

Title, *authors, meeting name, city, state, dates.

X. *Personal references* (if listed should number at least three)

(Name)
(Professional or business address)
(Phone)
(FAX)

There are firms available whose specific function is to compose and print CVs for professionals. Consult the Yellow Pages or physician journals for such listings. You may elect to use one of these services, but anyone with a physician's intelligence should certainly be capable of composing an appropriate CV following the guidelines in this chapter. The ability to compose the CV on a home computer, especially using a word processing program, is very helpful but not necessary. You can certainly compose a more than adequate CV with just a typewriter. The advantages of a computer-printer system include the ease with which revisions and additions of new information can be made, as well as the ability to run off multiple original copies of the CV (which are more impressive than photostatic copies).

If you are a generally poor speller or if English is not your native language, then you should enlist the aid of someone with good composition skills to edit the CV carefully once it is composed. A well-composed, well-organized, complete, but concise CV will impress those reviewing it with your organizational skills and your serious interest in the position being offered. In contrast, a poorly prepared, incomplete, or disorganized CV will likely lead the reviewer to attribute these same negative characteristics to you.

GENERAL RULES WHEN PREPARING A CV

1. Prepare a separate cover letter for each position for which you are applying.
2. Make sure all of your major accomplishments are listed accurately and completely.
3. Do not embellish, exaggerate, or analyze aspects of your history.
4. Be honest, thorough, complete, accurate, and concise.
5. Make sure an activity is listed for each major time period of your professional career (do not leave any "gaps" in the time frame of your upper educational and professional years). Do not include large volumes of unnecessary detail. Well-written CVs generally are 2–10 typewritten pages, with most CVs from residents being 2–5 pages in length.
6. Don't include too much detail about activities or awards before you went to college. By the time you become a medical professional, this information is pretty much irrelevant to most prospective employers.

There are quite a number of acceptable formats for arranging the text of your CV. A generic sample CV is given in Table 3.1. You certainly do not need to follow this format exactly, but this type of format is typical for CVs as used in academic institutions. A format to particularly avoid, however, is one organized by successive years (such as 1960 graduated from high school, 1964 graduated from college, 1968 graduated from medical school . . .). Following the career of someone who has written his or her CV in this fashion can be very tedious. The additional text of this chapter, following the sample CV (Table 3.1), discusses each portion of the CV in sequence. Items marked with an asterisk on the sample CV (Table 3.1) are optional.

Discussion of the Sample CV

An option on the first page of the CV is to place your name, contact address, and phone number at the top or upper corner of the CV so it is readily available. If you do not put it at the top of the first page, be sure to include it prominently in Section I, the Personal Data section at the beginning of the CV. Listing your main hobbies is usually appropriate or if you have interest in nonmedical applications skills. Do not overdo this section, however, because the reviewer is not evaluating you for your extracurricular interests, but for your professional qualities.

Under language fluency, you should probably only list a language if you are truly fluent in it. State something like "minimal fluency" or "able to write only" for languages in which you are not truly fluent. If you are applying surreptitiously (without the knowledge of your current employer), do not list the office telephone number in this first section of your CV.

In Section II, the Education section, listing any training before high school generally is neither important nor relevant. An exception might be some particular kind of relevant technical training before or in conjunction with high school. In listing the years of attendance in high school and college, you should write this as 1980 to 1983 or June 1980 to July 1983. Awards in this section should include only the major or medically relevant awards (further detail of the awards is not necessary in this section).

Section III, on Preresidency Professional Experience, obviously, could be left out if you did not have any sort of medical experience before becoming a physician. Appropriate things to list in this section are experiences as a volunteer worker, orderly or nurses' assistant, ambulance attendant or emergency medical technician, tutor for medical/paramedical students, research technician, or a worker for a medical subspecialty. It would also be appropriate to list nonmedical experience if it has relevance to medicine; however, listing of strictly business jobs without medical relevance would not be necessary or appropriate.

Section IV, Medical Practice Experience, would be left out if you have not had any practice experience outside of your residency program. However, if you did moonlight as a resident or did other kinds of medically pertinent work during residency, it would be appropriate to list these here. This section should also be used, of course, to list the medical positions held since finishing residency. Generally, these are most easily read if listed in order from past to present. If you are an emergency physician, Section IV could be retitled Emergency Medicine Experience. Sequentially listing the different institutions at which you have practiced in the Emergency Department would be appropriate. This could include the different hospitals in which you rotated as part of your residency program, as well as any places where you moonlighted. In addition, listing the number of airplane or helicopter transports in which you participated, if any, would be appropriate in this section. Any volunteer physician work, such as practice with free clinics or homeless clinics, would certainly be appropriate to list here. Additionally, any foreign or overseas medical experience or any separate military medical experience should be listed separately.

In Section V, under Current Professional Activities, you should list only those activities with significant relevance toward medicine. Under Committees and Appointments, it would be appropriate, in some cases, to list certain kinds of community service organizations, but do not overdo this. A listing of some recent Continuing Medical Education (CME) activities (such as conferences attended or ongoing CME programs by mail) may be appropriate to add at the end of this section. However, most potential employers do not want to wade through a complete list of all the CME activities you have done for the last 15 years; therefore, including only the most recent or prominent activities would be appropriate. Five or six activities are generally sufficient to list. Supplemental to your CV, however, you should probably prepare a formal list of all of your CME activities over at least the previous 3 years because this information is sometimes required for licensure or hospital privileges.

In Section VI, under Medical Licensure, you should list all of your current, active, state medical licenses and any other relevant licenses you possess. Including your Drug Enforcement Administration (DEA) number is optional, although at some point, this information would be required and verified by your potential employer.

Under Certification, the Board Certification section is very important. Board certification is becoming more and more important for hospital privileges as well as for various forms of licensure. If you are not yet board certified, you should certainly note in this section if you are eligible to take the boards or are already involved in the formal examination application process. Whether to put your actual board examination scores is optional; however, if your scores were exemplary, it certainly would not hurt to add them at this point. If, based on your board certification, you have been elected a fellow of a medical specialty organization or college, this should be denoted along with the relevant dates. Under Other Certifications, if you are certified ACLS, ATLS, PALS, APLS, or others, these should be clearly noted. A current certificate in these subjects is often required by various institutions, as well as by regional medical organizations. If you passed the National Board of Medical Examiners' examination or the Federal Licensing Examination (FLEX), you should denote that here along with your certificate number and the certification date.

Sections VIII and IX, on Publications and Presentations, are of key importance for academic positions and significantly less important for private practice positions. However, if you have relevant medical publications, these may help in applying for a private practice position as well. Generally, in Section VIII you should not include nonmedical publications unless you have reason to believe that they may be relevant or important to a potential employer. In the Presentations section, you should list only presentations to major regional, national or international medical meetings. You should generally not include simple lecture presentations to medical students or residents at your primary institution.

Opinions differ as to whether to include Personal References with your routine CV. Many believe that its inclusion is preferable in that it assures the reviewer that you have a number of reliable references. Before listing individuals, contact them about their willingness to serve as a reference for you (you should know that they will actually give you a good evaluation). If you are applying for a position without the knowledge of your present supervisor, leaving the references out might be appropriate as you would not want them contacted prematurely. However, for most applications, having the reference list already available for the prospective employer demonstrates your sincerity in looking at the position, and may also impress him or her with your reliability at having already obtained references. The optimal number of references varies from application to application. Generally, you should have at least three but probably not more than ten. In selecting your references, the most prominent or well-known members of your specialty from whom you can receive favorable, convincing recommendations are better than lesser known individuals or residents with whom you have worked. If you have spent significant time at a number of different institutions, you should generally have at least one major reference from each institution (rather than clustering all your references from a single institution).

The CV should routinely *leave out* the following information:

1. Religion (especially if it might affect your working hours);
2. Your sexual preference;
3. Personal health problems;
4. Disabilities;
5. Particular reasons you may have left certain positions in the past (this information could be relayed at the interview stage of an application).

In general, the CV should be organized in a fashion similar to that shown in Table 3.1 with the different sections clearly titled and denoted. When so arranged, it will not be necessary to underline, highlight, or change printing color to emphasize strong points of your application.

Cover Letter

In composing your cover letter, the following information should be included:

1. A brief statement indicating why you are interested in the particular position or outlining how the position fits your career goals.

2. Restate the address and phone number at which you can be reached (with a FAX number, if appropriate).
3. Indicate whether or not your current employer is aware that you are applying for this position and whether he may be contacted at this point.
4. A brief statement about particularly strong points of your curriculum vitae may, at times, be appropriate, but such a statement has to be carefully worded so as not to sound ostentatious.
5. If anything is deliberately left out of your CV, such as the reference list, you should note the reasons in the cover letter.

You should generally compose a new cover letter for each position for which you will be applying. Word the letter in such a way that the person reading it will think that it was meant uniquely for him or her. If properly constructed, your CV will not require alterations for submission for different positions.

INTERVIEW PROCESS

Preparing for a Job Interview

The first thing to consider is making sure you have an appropriate wardrobe for a job interview. Most medical professionals expect interviewees to wear a business-type suit. If you do not have one in your wardrobe, you probably should go ahead and purchase one in the last year of your residency. Certainly, the suit does not have to be expensive or of the latest style; in fact, an overly ostentatious suit tends to put off most potential interviewers. Generally, lightweight or medium-weight suits are best for interviews inasmuch as you do not want to get overheated or sweaty in a heavy wool suit during your interview.

You should also consider your hairstyle and how it might be interpreted by the interviewer. Generally, a particular hairstyle has minimal impact on most interviewers, but if you are a little shaggy, perhaps getting a haircut before the interview might be helpful. If you will be at an interview for more than 1 day or if you are going on several different interviews on the same trip, you should bring at least a second (and possibly a third) suit. This would allow you to change into a clean suit should you spill something during one of the early interviews or associated meals.

The other major concern before an interview is to consolidate and study the appropriate written materials in relation to the interview. This involves making sure your CV is up to date and that you bring several copies of it with you (in case one of your interviewers does not have a copy of it). You should carefully study your CV to know exactly what information is in it and on what pages the information is contained in case you are asked specific details about your CV. If you are applying for an academic position, it might also be helpful to bring reprints or copies of some articles you have published or copies of ongoing grant contracts that you hold. For some interviews it may be required that you send in ahead of time or have available all the documents verifying your training and licensing. This is covered in more detail in Chapter 5. Some of these documents may require certification by a notary public, so you should be sure to arrange this ahead of time.

You should have reviewed any readily available information about the position for which you are applying before the interview. Demonstrating to the interviewer that you have acquainted yourself with the position, to the extent possible, demonstrates your interest in the position and your planning skills. If information is readily available about the interviewer, knowing something about his or her background may prove useful during the interview and is worth reviewing ahead of time. It is often helpful to prepare a list of specific questions clarifying such points as benefits, work hours, and call responsibilities. This helps to ensure that you will not forget to ask key questions during the interview.

In general, you should make an effort to arrive at least 15 minutes early at the interview site or office. When being interviewed to join a clinic or office practice, arriving early is very helpful in that it allows you to observe the interactions of the office staff before your interview. One mundane but important piece of advice is to find a restroom so that you do not have to face the interview with a full bladder. This, of course, would also give you the opportunity to recomb your hair and otherwise straighten up. If you are already nervous, you might want to turn down any offers of coffee from the office staff if the caffeine might make you even more jittery. If lunch or another meal is part of the interview, be careful not to order anything with a high "spill potential," (such as a thick hamburger or spaghetti). Do not order the most expensive thing on the menu even if someone else is paying for the meal. It is probably best to avoid ordering wine or beer for lunch but would be okay for an evening meal if everyone else at the meal will be having alcoholic drinks.

Generally, the initial interview is mainly for exchange of information between the applicant and the recruiting practice. The important thing for you to explore during the initial interview is how you would fit into and enjoy the practice long-term rather than concentrating on some of the finer points such as specifics of the finances of the practice. Hammering out specific agreements regarding salary, benefits, and work schedules is generally done at a second or third interview, later in the acceptance process. Remember that everyone at the initial interview is usually on their very best behavior. Should you perceive a personality or interactive problem in the interview session, it is likely that this problem will be even worse in the future.

When joining a smaller group practice, it is very important to meet all of the members of the practice or the people who will be your main partners at the initial interview. When joining a larger clinic or multispecialty group practice, it is obviously not possible to meet everyone in the practice at the initial interview. However, when dealing with a smaller group it is very important initially to make certain that you seem to be generally compatible with each member of the practice. Consider asking the following questions at the initial interview.

I. Practice Structure

1. How is coverage on nights and weekends handled by the group?
2. How will this coverage be altered if you join the practice?
3. Is there any backup availability of other members of the practice?
4. What are the sources of referral for patients referred to the practice?
5. What are the consultant arrangements or availability of consulting staff for patients in the practice?
6. What limitations are there on referral of the patients to consultants?
7. How are new patients entering the practice delegated or assigned?

8. What percentage of the new patients, and what types of new patients will you receive?
9. What are the plans for future expansion of the group or practice?

II. Financial

1. What are the expected financial arrangements (i.e., what is the base salary, percent of gross practice income, or guaranteed hourly income that you will receive)?
2. What are the specific benefits provided, i.e., health insurance, dental insurance, life insurance, disability insurance (including the specific provisions and start time of the disability insurance), continuing medical education allotment, books and/or equipment?
3. What is the vacation time allotment and arrangements (i.e., how much vacation can be taken at one time, how is vacation time scheduled)?
4. How much sick leave is there and does it accumulate?
5. Will you receive any additional benefits or remuneration beyond your base salary (that is, will you receive a percentage of billings generated above your base salary)?
6. Are there any specific practice costs you will be expected to pay (such as providing any expenses or benefits for office staff)?
7. Does the practice have any other income-producing assets, such as x-ray, laboratory, associated physical therapy, occupational therapy facilities?
8. How is the extra income from these other sources divided in the practice?
9. Are there any additional bonuses paid within the practice and how are these determined?
10. Can you audit the books, or what are the specific audit ing arrangements of the practice finances?
11. Is there any allowance for travel expenses, moving expenses, or expenses involved in a second interview including your spouse?

III. Questions on job security and privileges

1. Can you be fired from the practice without written notice or what is the specific notification period required before you could be fired?
2. Based on what criteria could you possibly be fired?

3. Do you need to be board-certified to become a partner in the practice?
4. Can you pursue outside medical activities, such as a teaching affiliation with a residency program or medical school, working at a free clinic, doing lectures to medical groups or public organizations, or doing research or writing?
5. If there is any income from these activities, would this remain yours or would it have to be divided among the group?
6. Are there any special meetings or other organizations which you would be required to attend beyond those needed to retain hospital privileges?
7. What additional responsibilities would be expected of you outside of the practice?
8. How will the practice market or publicize your arrival?
9. Is there provision for a "testing out" or "breaking in" period to verify your compatibility in the practice?
10. Is there a "no competition" clause in the practice agreement (which would limit your ability to start a new practice after leaving the current one)?
11. How are the office staff hired, and what is the stability of the office staff?
12. Will you have any initial say in office staff hiring/firing and/or procedures?
13. What will be your allocation of office space and equipment?
14. What new equipment that you may require would the practice be able to purchase?

Make sure that all your important questions have been answered during the interview process. You should also ensure that your tour of the office or practice facility covers everything that you wanted to see.

After the Interview

If, after the interview, you are very interested in the practice opportunity, you should send thank-you notes to each of the major physicians involved in your interview. The notes should be relatively short and cordial, but should indicate your strong interest in the position. If, after the interview, you are not interested in pursuing the position, you should still send a thank-you note but only to the principal physician involved, and this note should not mention any future pursuit of the position.

On a second or follow-up interview, you should develop more in-depth questions about the finances and structure of the practice and should have clear in your mind what points you would like included in your contract with the group or practice. Your spouse or significant other should, of course, accompany you at the second interview, and arrangements should be made for your spouse to meet either some people within the practice or people within the community, as well as have a tour of the community or real estate market.

In interviewing for an academic medical position, you should try to meet some faculty members outside of the department to which you are applying. You should access some of the other departments' opinions of the physicians with whom you will be working. In addition, it would probably be helpful to talk to some of the residents in training at the institution to get their opinions on the interactions with the faculty. For an academic position, additional questions to be addressed include the following ones:

1. What are the patient care responsibilities of faculty versus residents (i.e., who writes orders, who performs specific major procedures, who handles follow-up and referrals)?
2. What are your specific requirements regarding participation in research and grant activities?
3. What are your specific teaching requirements in terms of hours and schedules?
4. What support facilities are available for teaching activities, i.e., secretarial staff for typing, running MedLine searches, obtaining books from the library, and assisting with research projects and grant application?
5. What are the physical facilities that the department has access to for teaching and research, i.e., biomedical photography, printing, statistical analysis, and computers?
6. What are the specific criteria used to determine faculty advancement and salary increases?
7. What are the evaluation procedures for residents and what evaluation is there of the faculty by the residents?

8. How does the department interact with the other departments in terms of referral, performing specific procedures, and division of training responsibilities?

Usually at the second interview a decision will be made to hire you or you will be in final competition with only a couple of other individuals for the position. At this interview, emphasize your strong points if there is still competition for the position; otherwise the interview would mainly be to iron out details of reimbursement and work or practice requirements. Before making final plans to accept any offer or position, you should make sure that a formal written agreement is available. A major decision such as this should not be made on the basis of verbal promises only. Chapter 4 discusses how to evaluate job offers and contracts.

Chapter 4

Evaluating Job Offers and Contracts

GOALS

The goals of this chapter are to present the specific items to include in an employment contract and to outline points of negotiation for a contract.

SECOND INTERVIEW

In general, any firm or group of physicians seriously evaluating you as an applicant will have you return for a second interview if they decide to offer you the position. At this time, you should determine if you are now the only candidate to whom the position is being offered or if you are still in competition with one or two other individuals. All of the considerations detailed in the previous chapters regarding preparation for the interview still apply. At this second interview, you need to prioritize your information-gathering to cover any specifics about the practice and its finances that were not covered at the first interview. Also, the fine points of your starting date and initial duties with the practice will need to be detailed. At the second interview, your spouse or significant other should accompany you, and the "host" physicians should have arranged some type of activities for your spouse (such as touring the community with a real estate agent or the spouse of one of the physicians, reviewing employment opportunities in the community with an employment officer, having interviews with school officials and/or local social organizations).

At the second interview, you should have a written list of specific features or negotiating points that you wish covered in the formal contract with the practice. Be certain that the following points are covered in the contract:

1. What is the start date for both work and office occupancy?
2. Will you have any phase-in of responsibility or clinical duties?
3. Is there a closing date to the agreement, or is there a specific date upon which contract renewal or change in your status with the practice will be renegotiated?
4. What is the length of the notification period (usually at least 4 weeks and sometimes up to 90–180 days) for termination of the employment agreement by either yourself or the practice?
5. Are there any penalties involved for canceling the agreement without due notice?
6. Are you allowed any employment opportunities outside the practice or are you permitted to do other related medical work (such as free clinic work, medical lecturing, involvement with a medical education program)?
7. Are there any specific criteria for which your employment would be terminated or for which your contract would not be renewed?
8. How will you be paid—salary, percent of gross billing, direct fee-for-service, other methods—and are there any other mechanisms in the practice for additional income?
9. What specific additional benefits are to be paid by the practice for you—employer social security, federal income tax, state income tax, local business tax, Worker's Compensation insurance, malpractice insurance, professional society dues, continuing medical education costs, health insurance, disability insurance, life insurance, retirement plan contributions, medical journal subscriptions, hospital staff fees, American Medical Association dues, other professional society dues, office equipment and supplies (disposable or reusable supplies), secretarial support services, vehicle and/or travel expenses?
10. What is the amount of vacation time allowed and what amount of this time may be taken continuously or as a single block?
11. Is there any additional allowance for sick leave time and/or continuing medical education (CME) or conference time?
12. Is there any "covenant to not compete" clause to prevent you from leaving the practice and going right into your own practice in the same community or vicinity?

13. Is there any specific timetable for a "buy in" plan to undertake partnership or part ownership of the practice?
14. How will the financial and payment arrangements change if and when you become a partner or part owner?
15. What specific office space will you be allocated and what will your abilities be to utilize the other office and support space owned by the practice?
16. What are the responsibilities of the office staff toward you in relation to the other practice members or physicians?
17. What will be your specific on-call duties and division of work responsibilities with the other members of the practice?
18. Will you be expected to contribute to buying any future equipment or property for the practice?
19. How are the assignments of patients distributed within the practice, how are new patients assigned to practice members, and how are referrals from other physician groups handled?

Some noncontractual considerations to evaluate further on your second interview include the following items:

1. Is the office space and equipment that you will be allocated sufficient for your needs?
2. Is there space for further growth in the practice and is the practice allowing for potential growth that you may cause by joining it?
3. Are the office personnel receptive toward you as an addition to the practice?
4. Does the practice own its office space and the facilities or are they leased? If leased, what is the long-term stability of the leasing arrangement?
5. Is there a great age difference between you and the members of the practice, and do you share any common interests with them outside of medicine?
6. Does the practice seem interested in adding you as a full-fledged partner in the future or just as a working employee?
7. Last, but perhaps most importantly, does your spouse or significant other seem happy with the choice of practice and community location?

If your second interview is to serve as a negotiating session about the specifics of your contract, then you should probably have a letter of intent in hand at the beginning of the interview. This letter of intent is a relatively brief document more or less written in nonlegal terms and is the document upon which the more formal contract can be based. If you follow the guidelines of the sample letter at the end of this chapter (Appendix 4.1), you should not need to involve a lawyer in composing the letter of intent. It is recommended that you obtain the services of an experienced contract lawyer to review your formal written contract with the practice before you sign it. Be certain to determine the lawyer's potential charges for this service before retaining him or her to review the contract.

Remember the following general principles of negotiation when hammering out the specifics of your contract:

1. Take the attitude that you want to be fair about the negotiations.
2. Don't bring up any surprises, hidden agendas, or misinformation during the negotiations.
3. Ask for everything you want at the beginning of the negotiations. (Don't bring up new major demands late in the negotiations.)
4. Don't let yourself be forced into signing a contract in haste or before you have had a chance to review it with your lawyer.
5. Make sure that all of the major clauses in your letter of intent are described in detail in the contract.
6. Expect that you will need to compromise at least on some minor points (the most stable and satisfactory contracts are ones in which each side feels they have gained something from negotiation).

BASIC ELEMENTS OF A CONTRACT

This section will review some of the basic elements in the composition of a formal contract. The term "contract" is defined as an agreement that creates an obligation. To be a contract, this agreement must bind the parties listed in the contract to perform certain acts.

Elements of a Binding Contract

There are several elements required of a binding contract:

1. Each party to the contract must be "competent." This entails that both parties are capable of understanding and appreciating the consequences of the specifics of the contract. When

you are dealing with a corporation, partnership or agency, you must be certain that the other party actually has the authority to offer and enforce the terms of the contract.

2. Mutual assent—simply, a mutual agreement on the terms of the contract. This basically takes the form of an offer by one side or the other (usually both, at different places in the contract) and an acceptance of that offer by the other party.
3. Legality—the terms of a contract must not violate any preexistent state, local, or federal law or regulation.
4. Good faith and lack of unconscionability—a contract imposes an obligation of good faith in its performance or enforcement on both parties. Unconscionability is a term describing a grossly oppressive, unfair, or outrageous clause in a component of the contract. If, on review of a contract, a court determines that a clause is unconscionable, then that portion of the contract is not enforceable or binding.

Legal Defenses

There are certain specific legal defenses under which a person may refuse to complete or carry out the terms of a contract. These include the following situations:

1. Fraud—defined as an intentional "perversion of truth" to induce one party to carry out a contract term or surrender a legal right.
2. Mistakes—some unintentional act, omission, or error arising from ignorance, surprise, or misplaced confidence. A mistake exists when a person (under some erroneous conviction of law or fact) does or omits to do, some act which, but for erroneous conviction, he or she would not have done or omitted.
3. Duress—defined as undue coercion or constraint to induce one party to act in a manner in which he or she would not otherwise act.
4. Illegality—that which is contrary to the principles of law. When a contract violates preexistent law, it is not enforceable.
5. Impossibility—this type of finding might occur if the terms required an unreasonable number of hours or other direct impairment of a physician's professional abilities such that to actually carry out the terms would be clearly impossible.

6. Frustration of purpose—when circumstances or events change such that the object of performance or purpose no longer exists, this aspect of the contract is no longer valid.
7. Statute of limitations—to enforce the penalty terms of a contract for one party not carrying out his or her obligations, this would have to be brought up in court within the declared statute of limitations (which varies from state to state). In general, the statute of limitations is anywhere from 2–6 years for written contracts.

Additional Cautions

There are additional contractual items of which to be wary:

1. Restrictions that would adversely impair the good practice of medicine (these would include such things as automatic consults to the senior physician in the group, requiring specific clearances from senior practice members for other consultations).
2. Any monetary "kick-back" requirements for referral physicians (remember that all forms of fee-sharing or fee-splitting in a referral situation are expressly prohibited by federal law).
3. Conflicting language in different sections of the contract document regarding the provisions of funds for salary or distribution.

Specific Headings

The specific headings to utilize in an employment contract include:

1. Purpose of the Letter of Intent or Contract (employer/employee relationship versus partnership, other; identity of the parties involved—list specific names and addresses)
2. Term of Contract (including time of any phase-in to employment or partnership)
3. Base salary/other financial arrangements
4. If salary is dependent upon any production or performance incentives
5. Vacation time
6. Continuing medical education time

7. Benefits
   A. Malpractice insurance
   B. Disability insurance
   C. Life insurance
   D. Health insurance
   E. Hospital dues
   F. Medical society dues
   G. Specialty association dues
   H. Pager
   I. Book allowance
   J. Travel
   K. Office supplies
   L. Expenses (meals when on duty, any others)

8. Practice coverage
   A. Office time
   B. On-call time
   C. Duties outside of patient care

9. Contingencies
   A. Privileges
   B. Licensure

10. Escape clauses
11. Causes for employment termination
    A. Illness
    B. Disability
    C. Failure to meet practice criteria
    D. Other

12. Covenants not to compete
13. Access to patient records/files
14. Dates or intervals when contract will be reviewed and by whom
15. Dates or intervals when contract is to be renewed and by whom
16. Details of entrance into practice
    A. Announcement cards
    B. Open House/party
    C. Business cards

   D. Stationery
   E. Name on office door or building sign
   F. Name in Yellow Pages

17. Outside income allocation
18. Call schedule
19. Voice in administration of the practice
    A. Hiring office staff
    B. Obtaining additional equipment
    C. Hiring additional physicians

20. General outline of partnership
    A. Time frame
    B. Equipment
    C. Satellite office/other facilities
    D. Buy in/buy out
    E. Right of first refusal
    F. Buy-back
    G. Disability or death of practice owner(s)

21. Date specified for the practice agreement to be written, signed and enacted

REVIEWING YOUR WRITTEN CONTRACT

Once the practice has drawn up a formal written contract for you to sign, you should carefully review it with your lawyer. One way to do this is to take a piece of paper and draw a line down the center and, on one side, list your obligations, and on the other side, list the obligations of the hiring practice. If the contract is one that is generally favorable to you, the two lists should either be about the same length or the list should be longer on the side of the practice obligations. Cross-reference the specifics of the contract to the above list provided in this chapter to make sure that all of the important points are covered. Remember when reading the contract that any statements using the verbs "may," "to the extent possible," "perhaps," or "under certain circumstances" are soft or "hedged" enough that they do not guarantee performance of whatever else is in the sentence. To make sure that promises in the contract will be carried out, the statements should include the words "shall," "must" or "will."

If, after reviewing the contract, you find any significant errors, omissions, or points that you think are different from the agreement reached, you should phone the practice's contact person and discuss it with him or her by phone. If the problem is easily resolved over the phone, then it will save you both some significant trouble in redrafting the contract. After you sign it, you should make a copy of the contract before sending it back to the practice for signature to guarantee that there are no alterations performed in it after you have signed it. Take the signing of a contract seriously because you may have very significant liabilities should you violate the terms of the contract in the future. One point to remember about the malpractice insurance coverage in your contract is to denote whether the specific policy utilized is a claims made or occurrence policy. If the policy is a claims made policy, then it should be specifically stated how the "tail" coverage will be paid if you leave the practice.

There are some additional considerations that apply to contracts for emergency medicine positions somewhat more than for other types of positions:

1. How many shifts per month are assigned?
2. What length of shift the physician will be expected to work?
3. How the shift schedule is derived and how far in advance the shifts are scheduled?
4. What flexibility there is to change shifts or trade them with other members in the group?
5. Under what circumstances can a patient's care be "signed out" to the next physician at the end of your shift and what is the mechanism of the "sign out" or care transfer?
6. Are the costs of specific required courses, such as ACLS, ATLS, prehospital radio control, and others, covered by the hospital or group?
7. Who actually has control over the terms of the contract, physician hiring, and employment termination, i.e., the hospital administrator or the members or director of the emergency physicians' group?
8. What will be the specific clinical responsibilities outside of the Emergency Department, i.e., managing emergencies on the inpatient side of the hospital, writing orders on admitted patients, "courtesies" to the hospital staff (e.g., inserting nasogastric tubes or Foley catheters on inpatients and reading

x-rays and ECGs on "off hours") or involvement with prehospital care systems?

9. What is the distribution within the practice group of night shifts, weekend shifts, and holiday shifts and how are these divided?
10. Are you required to "make up" any shifts missed due to vacation, illness, CME conference, etc.?

After the second interview process, it is hoped that you will have a number of different job offers or potential positions. It is certainly acceptable and to your advantage to somewhat play one off against the other if you are really uncertain as to which one might be the best for you. When telling one practice about the offers made to you by another practice, you should certainly be honest in providing them comparison information. Remember, however, that in certain specialties there are a large number of applicants, and if you are too adamant or demanding in your contract negotiations, the practice may offer the position to another equally qualified candidate. It is to your advantage to actually follow all the way through to the second interview stage with several different practices, especially if they are in the same geographic area, just to make sure that the salary and benefits you are being offered at any one of these practices are consistent with the norm for the region.

Appendix 4.1 is a sample letter of intent, originally published and copyrighted by the Pennsylvania Medical Society. This shows an example of the wording of letters of intent or contracts applicable to most private practice situations. A substantial part of this sample letter is material related to considerations involving eventually becoming a partner or part owner of a practice. The letter can obviously be shorter where these conditions are not applicable (such as when you are to remain an employee or contractor). The sample letter of intent also contains a "covenant to not compete" clause, which is not a part of all physician contracts. For example, seldom would a "covenant to not compete" clause be acceptable for individual contracts with hospital-based physicians such as emergency physicians. However, some hospital contracts have utilized this type of clause to prevent radiologists or pathologists from leaving a hospital and setting up a competing radiology or laboratory service near the hospital.

A signature by a witness (attesting to the authenticity of the signature of the person(s) signing the contract) is not usually necessary for a medical contract. However, it may be advisable under some circumstances to have a contract signed in the presence of a notary public for signature verification. This service usually only costs about $5.00–10.00 and can usually be performed by the lawyer whom you have retained to review the contract.

SAMPLE LETTER OF AGREEMENT[a]

Letter of Agreement for physician employment between _______ (practice name) and _______ (individual's name) _______ , M.D.

Dear Dr. _______ :

As we have discussed at our meetings of _______ (date) and _______ (date), this letter is intended to set out our agreement for your initial employment with our practice. We hope it will be useful in making clear the suggested details of our relationship. Your employment is, of course, contingent upon your obtaining active staff privileges at _______ (hospital) and courtesy staff privileges at _______ hospital and a valid _______ (state) license to practice medicine, all prior to _______ (date). If it meets with your approval, we would appreciate you signing this letter and two copies of it and returning them to us at your earliest convenience. The details will, of course, be reduced to a more formal employment agreement (if you desire), and they may have to be so drafted by our attorney to meet our professional corporation requirements. We are, however, satisfied to let this informal, but legally binding, letter set forth our understanding. It will certainly determine the terms of any more formal document.

1. You will be an employee of our medical practice (corporation) for _______ months starting _______ , (date) 19___ . While only that relationship is described in this letter, we have discussed our plans for a future relationship and are entering a separate letter of agreement as to the specifically agreed ongoing details. No assurance can be made by either of us, at this time, that we will proceed past _______ , 19___ , but if all circumstances are favorable to each of us, the _______ (discussed) (agreed) format (described in item 13 below) will become our arrangement starting _______ , 19___ . We propose to start discussions on this topic after

________ , 19 ___ , with a firm offer (if any) and decision to be made by ________ , 19___ .

In addition, either you or we may terminate this initial employment at any time within the ________ months' employment period on ___ days notice to the other. If we should terminate your employment during that time, your salary will continue for those ________ days or until you obtain other full-time employment or practice, if sooner.

2. As an employee, you will be involved full-time in our practice of ________ (medicine, surgery, etc.), and you will not take any outside medical practice employment during this period without written permission from us.
3. It is particularly important that both of us realize that the initial ________ months of your employment in the practice represents a trial period for us. During that time, you will be evaluating how you like working with us and with the practice. Similarly, we will be evaluating you and how you fit in with the practice. To this end, we hope you will be agreeable to having not only ________ (informal, formal) discussions as we go along, but also more formal regularly scheduled meetings for discussion every ________ months. We hope by this means we can make every effort to assure a highly successful relationship which will develop into a lasting arrangement.

During your employment period, in addition to your clinical competence, there are several specific items which we feel would be essential to your overall success and which we will evaluate. These are:

A. The commitment of your time
B. Your productivity and efficiency in handling patient matters
C. Your willingness and effectiveness in promoting the practice and yourself
D. Your acceptance by patients, physicians, and hospital personnel
E. Your acceptance of practice obligations and responsibilities
F. Your interest in the practice from an entrepreneurial standpoint
G. A clearly demonstrated ability for us to work together with good rapport and understanding

4. We propose a salary of $_______ which is $_______ per month for your initial _______ months' employment. If your employment continues, we will provide a salary of $ (an increase in salary of not less than $_______ for the next 12 months). For the remainder of your employment, we will provide an annualized salary of $_______ ($_______ per month).

In addition to the extent that our practice's "net income" (meaning the sum of salaries, bonuses, retained income and retirement contributions to or for _______ (us shareholders) (me as sole shareholder) (us partners) (me as sole owner) measured at each fiscal year end (_______) exceeds _______ (%, such as 105% or 110, etc.) of the comparable amount in the immediately preceding 12 months, you will be entitled to a portion of the excess as follows:

_______	___%
_______	___%
_______	___%

We are happy to share with you this above income above what we anticipate to be our "break even point" on your involvement.

In addition, the corporate Board of Directors occasionally declares and pays bonuses based upon individual merit and corporate results.

5. We delineate a "total compensation" package for you as follows:

You will be entitled to _______ (%) of collections for services personally rendered by you to be paid to you or on your behalf by the practice. The items to be paid include:

a. A monthly draw against compensation in the gross amount of $_______ (and to be adjusted from time to time as we agree);
b. Bonus (as applicable above);
c. All tax withholdings, Employer Social Security, FUTA taxes, and Worker's Compensation insurance;
d. Reimbursement of business expenses including (but not limited to) malpractice insurance, _______ (entertainment expenses, travel and educational expenses, professional society dues, etc.); and

e. The cost of corporate provided fringe benefits _______ (health, disability, and life insurance, retirement plan contributions) and the like which the corporation may from time to time provide in its benefit plans for employees and subject to the terms of those plans as adopted.

A reconciliation of the amounts paid to you or on your behalf with your retirement for "total compensation" will be made semiannually and any amounts due you paid within 30 days thereafter. Similarly, if you are for any reason overdrawn with respect to your entitlement, you will repay that amount to the corporation within 30 days of the determination and notice to you.

6. The practice (corporation) will also pay the cost of your professional liability insurance (currently _______ type of policy) and your professional society dues, journal subscriptions (up to $_______ per year), and hospital staff fees. In addition, we will pay you $_______ per month for business use of your automobile and we will pay or reimburse you for professional education and travel expenses up to $_______ per year. However, other practice-related expenses such as additional educational, automobile, entertainment, etc., costs will have to be paid out of your earnings during your employment period. We estimate the cost of the items provided by the practice for you to be $_______ during your first year.
7. Because we practice as a professional corporation, you will also be entitled to certain fringe benefits. These include our payment of _______ (Blue Cross/Blue Shield) (basic health) and major medical insurance for you and your family, group term life insurance protection of at least $_______, (in whatever amount is provided under any corporation plan we maintain,) and payment of reimbursement for disability insurance premiums for coverage of at least $_______ per month after a 90-day waiting period. We estimate that the package of fringe benefits for you will total about $_______ during your first year.

You have also stated your preference not be to covered by our _______ (pension plan), (profit sharing plan) (plans) in the _______, (months or year), even if you qualify to participate, and if necessary, you thus agree to sign a form so stating your waiver.

Our practice maintains a _______ (pension) (and profit sharing) plan. However, rules of this Internal Revenue Service approved plan require a waiting period of 36 months for entry into the plan. You will, therefore, receive your entire remuneration as salary for the period of _______ months that you are an employee of the practice. If you advance to co-ownership or partner status, however, these months spent as an employee will count toward the eligibility requirement for retirement contributions for you.

8. You will be entitled to _______ weeks' paid vacation during your first 12 months of employment and to _______ weeks of absence for educational and/or professional society meetings. You will be entitled to _______ weeks' paid vacation during the next 12 months (during the remaining _______ -month employment period) and to _______ additional week(s) of absence for educational and/or professional society meetings. Arrangements for all such absences must, of course, be made to assure that our practice is properly covered. Any unused absences cannot be carried over to succeeding years, nor will they be paid for.
9. In case of absence due to illness or injury, your basic salary will continue for a period not exceeding _______ days plus any unused vacation time. Absence in excess of that would be without pay.
10. During the initial _______-month employment period, you will not be required to contribute any money toward the practice's equipment or operations, but likewise, your work will give you no financial interest in the practice's accounts receivable, furniture, equipment, leasehold, patients' charts and records, and the like.
11. In the course of inviting you to practice with us in _______ (location) and in your employment, we will be introducing you to and making available all our contacts and referring doctor relationships, ongoing patient contacts, general hospital sources, and the like. We have discussed how termination of your employment for any reason of any manner followed by your practicing in the area would cause you to take many of those sources of our practice with you to our real detriment, for we would have established you in a situation that would make you a very strong competitor for our current and potential practice sources.

Therefore, you agree that you will not enter into the practice of _______ in any manner or capacity within a radius of _______ miles of any office then maintained by our practice corporation or within _______ miles of _______ hospital for at least _______ years if your employment terminates any time and for any reason even if we were to ask you to leave during the initial employment period in question or thereafter until and unless a succeeding written contract no longer contains such restrictions.

You expressly agree that the corporation is empowered to enforce this restrictive covenant by obtaining an injunction in a court of law or equity (without the necessity of posting any bond or cash or otherwise) and should the corporation obtain such an injunction then whatever portion of that _______-year period has not run as of the date the covenant was first violated shall extend the time the restrictive covenant will be effective upon you from the date of final adjudication of the claim for injunctive relief. That your violating this restrictive covenant will subject you to an agreed liability of $_______ payable to our corporation immediately upon such competitive practice as estimated damages for your action, (or that the court may determine suitable damage payment). If you fail or refuse to pay such amount, you also agree that the corporation may obtain a court injunction (without posting bond) to prevent your so practicing until the agreed sum is paid and that your violating it will subject you to an agreed liability payable to our corporation immediately upon such competitive practice as estimated damages for your action. We have discussed how the cumulative total compensation paid to or for you during the employment period would be a reasonable method of estimating the damages from such competition, since those monies paid in expectation of a continuing relationship would have instead staked you to a competitive position; hence the damages will be the sum of all gross salary payments, bonuses, fringe benefit costs and retirement plan contributions, if any, you have received from _______ (time or date) until the date of termination but not in excess of $_______. If you fail or refuse to pay such amount, you also agree that our corporation may obtain a court injunction (without posting bond) to prevent your so practicing until the agreed sum is paid.

12. Recognizing your duty to the corporation as an employer, you agree that if your employment terminates for any reason

or in any manner whether or not you practice within the restricted area as described above, you will in no event solicit, directly or indirectly, any patient (or member of any patient's immediate family) from the practice's services or solicit, directly or indirectly, any contractual arrangement of the ________ (corporation or practice) for a period of ________ years following termination of your employment.

13. In the event that during your employment period, we should die or become totally and permanently disabled from the practice of ________ (medicine, surgery) then you agree to purchase the practice (owned by our corporation) within days of the death or disability for an amount equal to the sum of (a) ________ % of the original cost of the equipment, furniture, and fixtures (excluding automobiles not included in this sale), (b) ________ % of the face amount of accounts receivable, (c) ________ % of the cost of medical supplies and inventories, and (d) ________ % of the most recent fiscal year's gross income. The purchase price is to be paid in equal monthly installments of principal over a ________-month period with monthly interest payments on the unpaid principal balance at the rate of ________ % annually and is to be represented by a promissory note signed by you (and your spouse). The purchase price is to be allocated among the assets of the practice as follows:

Equipment, etc.	as in (a) above
Accounts receivable	as in (b) above
Supplies and inventory	as in (c) above
Goodwill	___% of the remainder
Medical charts and records	___% of the remainder
Leasehold	___% of the remainder
Use of practice name for 2 years	___% of the remainder

14. If you and we agree to proceed in practice together after ________, 19___, we will sell you sufficient shares (a sufficient ownership interest) in our ________ (corporation, practice) for you to become an equal ________ (shareholder, partner). The price for ________ (those shares, that interest) will be based upon the ________ (corporation's, practice's) "net book value" (which would not include ________ (accounts receivable, automobiles, or goodwill) as

of ________, 19___, such figure to be modified so that depreciation on all equipment, furnishings, and fixtures (except for any automobiles) will be restated by using straight line depreciation over a ________-year useful life.

However, your purchase of our ________ (shares, interest) will be subject to our "Senior Doctor's Protection" in case of a split-up between us. This "Senior Doctor's Protection," in the form of a "Stock Option" ("Partnership Interest Option") give us the right to repurchase your shares (partnership interest) any time up to ________, 19___, and to thereby retain the practice, office, telephone numbers, etc. Our repurchase of your shares (partnership interest) would be at the same stock (partnership interest) valuation formula and terms as your initial purchase.

Furthermore, if you and we agree to proceed in practice together after ________, 19___, you will participate in the income sharing arrangement ________ (equal; productivity; or a combination of the two) that you and we agree to, except that your calculated share of such income, which would include ________ (salary, any bonuses, retirement plan contributions, and dividends plan, any retained corporate profit but less any corporations loss and any specially agreed "semipersonal expenses") will be multiplied by the following percentages to determine your "discounted" share of the practice's income:

During the fiscal year ending
________, 19___ = ___%
During the fiscal year ending
________, 19___ = ___%
During the fiscal year ending
________, 19___ = ___%
During the fiscal year ending
________, 19___ = ___%
After ________, 19___ = 100%

(reduced in each of the first ________ years of co-ownership by an amount equal to one-________ of the sum of ___ % of the outstanding practice accounts receivable as of ________ plus _____ % of the immediately preceding year's practice gross income.)

We hope this proposal meets with your approval, and we look forward to our working together starting ________, 19___. If you agree to these terms and agree that they will be legally binding upon you and us, please sign two copies of this letter and the enclosed two copies and return them to us. We will each then have copies signed by the other, evidencing our agreement.

As mentioned, if you want to discuss any parts of this proposal further, please give us a call at your earliest convenience.

Sincerely,
(CORPORATION NAME)
(By): ________ M.D./D.O.
(President)

Agreed and accepted this _______ day of _______ , 19___ .

____
(physician's name)

____
Witness signature

____
Date

[a]Reprinted with permission from the "Planning for Your Retirement" handbook, prepared for the Pennsylvania Medical Society by The Health Care Group, Plymouth Meeting, PA.

Chapter 5

Licensing and Obtaining Hospital Privileges

GOALS

The goals of this chapter are to present a timetable to follow in the last year of residency to prepare for medical practice, and to present the specific steps to follow to obtain a medical license and hospital privileges.

An important part of your practice planning is to obtain the appropriate medical licenses and hospital privileges needed for your private practice.

SUGGESTED TIMETABLE

The following is a suggested timetable to use in your last year of residency to plan and arrange your postresidency employment.

Twelve Months Before Start Date

1. Review the geographic areas in which you are interested with your spouse or significant other. Start the community selection process as detailed in Chapter 2.
2. Obtain maps and tourist bulletins of the areas in which you are interested.
3. Notify a few physician recruiter organizations about your areas of interest and start having them send you preliminary information on opportunities in those areas. (The use of recruitment firms, however, may make your application less attractive to some potential employers if payment of large recruitment fees becomes a condition of your employment.)

4. Start scanning the employment advertisements in the major journals of your medical specialty. Directly investigate any outstanding job opportunities. Even at this early date, you and the advertising practice may wish to make a commitment to each other.
5. Contact the state medical licensing board and request an application for a medical license (see Appendix 5.1 at the end of this chapter for the specific addresses for each state's licensing board and the requirements to obtain a license in each state).
6. Contact the telephone company in the communities in which you are interested to obtain information about a listing for the following year in the Yellow Pages.
7. Contact the appropriate local government organization to obtain information on getting a business license for that location.
8. Read this book carefully. Consider attending seminars on practice start-up and reviewing other written information on the general aspects of starting in medical practice.
9. If you are going to start a new practice, consider hiring a practice management consultant at this time to assist in setting up the practice.
10. With your spouse or significant other, decide upon the specific important items you would want included in your initial practice contract.
11. Write your CV and line up several potential faculty members or other physicians who could serve as personal references for your applications.
12. Buy a decent suit for interviews if you do not already have one.
13. Have some passport-sized photos of yourself taken so they will be quickly available if you need them for applications. These photos can be easily and inexpensively obtained at any American Automobile Association office.

Ten to Eleven Months Before Start Date

1. Identify a number of potentially interesting positions. Mail your CV and cover letter to these positions.
2. Start making "screening trips" to areas you are considering (perhaps in conjunction with vacation time), even if you do not have formal interviews there yet.

3. Utilize the secondary sources of information on practice opportunities listed in Chapter 1 (writing to the county medical society or chief of hospital staff, and others) if you have not yet identified any practice opportunities in which you might be interested.

Nine Months Before Start Date

1. At this point, try to narrow your choices of potential practices down to two or, perhaps, three sites.
2. Apply for a Federal DEA license if you do not already have one. Their mailing address is: U.S. Department of Justice, Drug Enforcement Administration, P.O. Box 28083, Central Station, Washington, DC 20005; 202–633–1000.
3. If you are going to be setting up your own office, begin specific searches (your spouse might have more time to do this) for office sites. At this point, this would entail contacting a local realtor, hospital administrator, or a leasing agent.

Six to Seven Months Before Start Date

1. If you are joining a group or practice already in existence, you should have a letter of intent from the group, if not a final contract, by this point.
2. Apply for hospital privileges.
3. Write the local county medical society for information on joining the society.
4. If starting your own practice, narrow your office site choices to two or three, and begin lease negotiations for the office site.
5. If you are building a new office, you should, at this point, have the office design completed and have a contract with a construction firm.
6. If you need a loan to start up the office, you should have applied for it by this time.
7. Order the furniture and equipment for your office.

Four to Five Months Before Start Date

1. Contact the malpractice insurance company that will be providing your malpractice insurance; make sure that you are appropriately registered with them, and fill out any paperwork required by them.

2. If you are building a new office, the actual construction should certainly have started by this point.
3. Arrange for printing of your office stationery, business cards, announcement cards, open house information, and patient information materials.
4. Contact the medical insurance agencies with whom you will be dealing (Blue Cross/Blue Shield, Medicaid, Medicare, and state Worker's Compensation insurance) to ascertain the proper paperwork required for registration with them.
5. Choose and order your office telephone equipment; make sure you are listed in the local Yellow Pages. Order any other office medical equipment necessary.
6. Order and organize the office paperwork and computer systems that you will need.
7. Once you have confirmed your practice address, obtain a Federal employer identification number (for tax purposes) from the Internal Revenue Service. You should apply through your local IRS office and request an SS-4 form.
8. Obtain a state employer identification number through the state employment office or labor department.
9. Contact the local city or county clerk's office to apply for any necessary occupancy permits or local business licenses.
10. Determine if a state narcotics license (separate from your federal DEA license and number) is required, and apply for one through the appropriate state agency.

Two Months Before Start Date

1. Make sure the office signs and labels have been ordered or made.
2. Prepare a procedure manual for your office (see Chapters 7 and 8).
3. Plan the staffing schedule.
4. Set your fee schedule.
5. Send out preliminary announcements to the local newspaper and county medical society newsletter about the start of your practice.
6. Talk to several moving companies, obtain moving cost estimates, and make preliminary arrangements for moving. If you will be hiring new employees, the advertisements should be placed by this time, and you should start interviewing

prospective employees (having this arranged even further in advance obviously is helpful).

7. Obtain the "Tax Guide for Small Business" book and payroll withholding booklets from the IRS.

One Month Before Start Date

1. Finish hiring your office staff.
2. Make sure all of the office paperwork and billing paperwork has arrived and is suitable.
3. Contact the local utilities companies to make sure your office utilities have been turned on.
4. Make sure the furniture and equipment has been delivered to the office and start arranging it.
5. Bond all the employees.
6. Try to meet some of the physicians and referral sources within the community as well as other people who will interact with the practice (hospital administrators, other facility administrators, and others). Attending the hospital's business meetings or teaching conferences (as your residency commitments allow) is a good way to meet referral sources.

Opening Week of Your Practice

1. Have additional announcements placed in the newspaper, newsletters, and possibly on local TV or radio about the practice opening.
2. Attend some local medical and civic meetings at which you may meet potential referral physicians and other referral sources.
3. Consider scheduling and advertising a "practice opening reception or party" to be held at your office.

OBTAINING PRIVILEGES

An important item when going into private practice is obtaining hospital privileges. This can be a lengthy process. The credentials committee of the hospital, whose approval is required to obtain privileges at the hospital, may only meet once every 2–3 months. The first step in obtaining hospital privileges is to contact the hospital medical staff office and obtain an application form to join the staff. Some hospitals may have an application fee or may require that you pay the first year's medical staff dues along with your application. To speed your application, be certain that you fill out all portions of the application completely. Send all of the additional documentation required, which usually includes copies of your DEA certificate, your medical school diploma, your National Board or FLEX certificate, your certificate of satisfactory completion of residency, your state license, letters of recommendation, and a document verifying that you have obtained appropriate malpractice insurance. You may need to have notarized copies of these documents obtained and sent from each relevant office.

At most hospitals, after review of all of this material by the credentials committee (which is composed of a number of physicians on the hospital's medical staff), the committee will invite you for a personal interview. This interview is often more extensive if you are applying for hospital privileges as a new solo practitioner. However, if you are joining a preexisting group, the credentials committee recognizes that the group itself should have reviewed your background very carefully, and the committee may essentially "rubber stamp" its approval for your hospital privileges. At the interview with the credentials committee, you should be prepared to answer any questions about the adequacy of your training, any "gaps" in your postgraduate time, any malpractice suits in which you have been involved and their outcomes, and specifically how you plan to interact with the physicians already on the hospital staff.

An important part of applying for hospital privileges is delineating specifically what procedures you wish to perform. Most credentials committees now look very carefully at this. For example, to apply for Swan-Ganz catheter insertion privileges and other invasive procedures, it is usually necessary that you demonstrate that you have received formal training in the performance of these, as well as documentation as to the number of these specific procedures you have performed in your residency. As part of credentialing, you may have to apply separately for ICU privileges, for hospital consultation privileges, and for privileges to admit patients to the hospital with consultation from other physicians. Be certain that the privileges you are applying for are as extensive and appropriate to your abilities as you require for your practice. Along with your application, the hospital medical staff office should send you copies of the hospital's bylaws and a specific delineation of your privileges. Be certain that you review these carefully before your interview so that you can utilize the interview to clarify any ambiguities in the hospital bylaws document or in the privileges which you have been granted or denied.

Often, to maintain hospital privileges you have to meet certain requirements, such as serving on hospital committees and attending specific hospital medical staff meetings. If you have a particular preference as to a specific hospital committee on which you wish to serve, you should inform the credentials committee at the time of the interview. As a new medical staff person, it may be best to avoid serving on a committee such as the credentials committee. The members of the credentials committee are often required to make decisions restricting a physician's practice; this could be politically difficult for you as a new physician in the community. Initially, serving on committees that have less controversial functions, such as the medical records committee or antibiotic review committee, might be politically safer.

Another important consideration is obtaining a federal DEA license. You will need at least an individual practitioner license to prescribe controlled substances in Schedules II–V. If you plan to have specific Schedule II–V drugs available in your office (for dispensing), you will need a separate office or institutional DEA number. Be certain that, if you are going to utilize in-office controlled substances, you comply very carefully with the demanding record-keeping and other DEA requirements regarding these substances.

To obtain a state medical license, you merely have to write to the state licensing office (see Appendix 5.2). There is now considerable reciprocity with regard to licensure among different states, and if you already have at least one state license, the process of obtaining a license in another state is often considerably simplified. For some state licenses, a personal interview is required, and you should plan your subsequent visits or vacation around this. You might need to utilize some of your vacation time to make the interview trip for the state license inasmuch as the interview for the license is often only held in the capital city of the state. In addition, to obtain a license in some states, a copy of a birth certificate, validated fingerprints, and other paperwork that you do not need for other medical applications may be necessary. Some states require that the verification of passing either the FLEX or National Board Exam be sent to them directly from the exam office, and they will not accept a copy of the exam certificate from you. At the conclusion of this chapter, a further listing of the endorsement and reciprocity policies of the state boards is presented.

The AMA publishes a book (revised annually) entitled, "U.S. Medical Licensure Statistics and Current Licensure Requirements, 1994 Edition." ($35 for members, $60 for nonmembers; you can order it by calling 1–800-621–8335; order #OP399091.)

Appendix 5.1

[a]Reprinted with permission of *Resident & Staff Physician*
May 1993 by Romaine Pierson Publishers, Inc.

How to Get Your License: A State-by-State Guide[a]

Here is all you need to know to become licensed to practice medicine in your own particular state, including how and when to apply for FLEX, the documents necessary for submitting an application, requirements needed to be accepted for the licensing exam, and where to call or write for more information.

THE FLEX

The Federation of State Medical Boards of the United States (FSMB) provides the Federation Licensing Examination (FLEX) and makes it available to all FSMB member licensing Boards. At the present time, medical licensing Boards of all states of the United States, the District of Columbia, Guam, Puerto Rico, and the Virgin Islands, as well as the Canadian province of Saskatchewan, use FLEX for licensure. Of the 15 separate osteopathic licensing Boards in the United States, all but Florida, Michigan, Nevada, Oklahoma, and West Virginia use or at least accept FLEX for licensure. Besides FLEX, certification of the National Board of Medical Examiners (NBME) or the National Board of Osteopathic Medical Examiners (NBOME) is accepted by most states in lieu of FLEX. *NBME certification alone is not accepted by the medical licensing Board of the Virgin Islands, nor is it available to graduates of medical schools not accredited by the LCME* (schools outside the United States and Canada). NBOME certification alone is not accepted for unrestricted licensure by the licensing Boards of Louisiana, Montana, North Carolina, and the Virgin Islands. The NBME Part I and Part II examinations have been replaced by Step 1 and Step 2 of the United States Medical Licensing Examination (USMLE).

The last administration of NBME Part III will be in May 1994. USMLE also replaces the present FLEX examination. The last FLEX examination for initial licensure will be administered in December 1993. *For information concerning Steps 1 and 2 of USMLE, please contact the USMLE Secretariat.*

• FLEX consists of two complementary components. FLEX Component 1 is designated to evaluate measurable aspects of knowledge and understanding of basic and clinical science principles and mechanisms underlying disease and modes of therapy most frequently encountered in a supervised practice setting. FLEX Component 2 is designed to sample the additional knowledge and cognitive abilities required of a physician delivering medical care in an independent practice setting.

• FLEX is given twice yearly, in June and December. Each component of FLEX is one and one-half days in length. In all states, a minimum score of 75 on each component is required for passing. Some states require that both components be passed in a single sitting. Others have sequence requirements, i.e., Component 1 must be passed before Component 2.

• In December 1991, 3,931 examinees took both components of FLEX: the pass rate was approximately 67%. In June 1992, 7,058 examinees took both components of FLEX; the pass rate was approximately 77%.

• FLEX eligibility requirements, application, deadlines, fees, etc., vary from state to state. See the state-by-state listing beginning on page 72 for information on your state. FLEX applications and more detailed information about state requirements should be obtained from the Board from which the license is being sought.

• Under the rules established by the Accreditation Council for Graduate Medical Education (ACGME), a foreign medical school graduate (FMG) must be certified by the Educational Commission for Foreign Medical Graduates (ECFMG) in order to be eligible for appointment to an accredited graduate medical education training program in the United States.

• To earn ECFMG certification, FMGs are required to pass a medical science examination (FMGEMS or Parts I and II of the NBME examination sequence or, now, Steps 1 and 2 of the USMLE) and the English language proficiency test administered worldwide by the ECFMG, and to document completion of the educational requirements to practice medicine in the country in which they have received their medical education. FMGEMS is designed to assess knowledge in the basic medical and clinical sciences. The exam is given in January and in July on two successive days. Registration for the FMGEMS and the ECFMG English Test closes three months before the date of the exam. The last administration of the FMGEMS will be in July 1993. Fees for 1993 are $275 for each day taken separately or $450 for both days and the English test. The fee for the ECFMG English test has increased to $30. ECFMG administers Step 1 and Step 2 of USMLE to foreign medical students and graduates. Step 1 was administered for the first time in June 1992 and Steps 1 and 2 in September 1992. For more information, please contact the Educational Commission for Foreign Medical Graduates directly.

- With the September 1989 administration, ECFMG accepted passage of NBME Parts I and II exams in lieu of FMGEMS for ECFMG certification.
- The majority of state Boards regulate the licensing of both M.D.s and D.O.s under one governing body. Thus, for those states, the process for unrestricted licensure of a D.O. is the same as for an M.D. However, the following states have separate governing Boards for D.O.s: Arizona, California, Florida, Hawaii, Maine, Michigan, Nevada, New Mexico, Oklahoma, Pennsylvania, Tennessee, Utah, Vermont, Washington, and West Virginia.

For further information on FLEX, contact:

Federation of State
Medical Boards
6000 Western Place, Suite 707
Fort Worth, TX 76107
(817) 735-8445

For further information on ECFMG certification, contact:

Educational Commission for
Foreign Medical Graduates
3624 Market Street
Philadelphia, PA 19104
(215) 386-5900

For more detailed information on individual state licensing requirements, write to the Board from which you want to obtain a license.

The National Boards

Certification by the NBME may be used as one avenue to licensure in the United States for those certified as diplomates prior to implementation of the United States Medical Licensing Examination (USMLE) and for examinees taking a combination of NBME and USMLE examinations prior to the year 2000, as described below. With the implementation of USMLE, the NBME has reaffirmed its commitment to issue its certificate based upon successful completion of USMLE Steps 1, 2, and 3 and any other requirements established and announced by the NBME.

With the phase-out of the NBME examinations, students who enrolled in U.S. medical schools in the fall of 1990 or later will use USMLE for purposes of licensure.

The last regular administrations of NBME certifying examinations are scheduled as follows:

Part I was given in September 1991

Part II was given in April 1992

Part III will be given in May 1994

Although many persons may already have successfully completed some part of a licensing examination sequence before the implementation of USMLE, only those who pass all three steps of USMLE will be reported to states as successfully completing the USMLE examination sequence. However, to ensure a fair opportunity for persons who have partially met examination requirements for licensure under the current systems, candidates for certification by NBME who have passed either NBME Part I or NBME Part II, but have not passed all three parts of the NBME certification examination prior to the phase-out, will be certified as NBME diplomates to state licensing Boards on meeting all nonexamination requirements and successfully passing a combination of Part I or Step I, Part II or Step 2, and Part III or Step 3.

Detailed information about the NBME and its examinations is provided in the Bulletin of Information 1993 on National Board Examinations and in the April 1993 Part II or 1993 Part III Examination General Instructions, Content Outline, and Sample Items. These annual publications are made available to all applicants from the National Board of Medical Examiners, 3930 Chestnut Street, Philadelphia, PA 19104 (215/590-9500).

Certification Activity—Based on current information provided by the states, National Board certification alone is recognized by the medical licensing authorities of all states and licensing jurisdictions *except the Virgin Islands.* Additionally, the certificate of the National Board is accepted for initial licensure in the Canadian provinces of Alberta and Ontario.

In 1991, the NBME certified 12,217 diplomates of the Board. The number for 1990 was approximately 12,418. In 1991, the number of endorsements of record of certification to state medical licensing boards requested by National Board diplomates was 25,360.

Part III of the National Boards—Part III, the final examination for National Board certification, is a one-day, written (multiple-choice) examination intended to measure a candidate's possession and use of medical knowledge that is deemed appropriate for the unsupervised practice of general medicine.

The content of Part III reflects a two-dimensional organization of clinical problems. First, problems are grouped by type of clinical encounter, which includes patient characteristics, care setting, acuity, and other characteristics. Second, problems are grouped according to an evaluative objective, which is associated with the physician task (that is, taking the history, prescribing pharmacotherapy, making referrals). The clinical problems encompass the full range of severity, from health maintenance to acute, multisystem problems with grave prognoses. The clinical problems also are related to ambulatory and hospital settings.

Description of the Examination—Some of the items refer to pictorial or graphic material that requires knowledge and skills related to patient management. For example, you may be asked to interpret roentgenograms, photomicrographs, sonograms, CT scans, and pictures of lesions, among others.

The items are written and reviewed by multidisciplinary committees made up of senior faculty members, teachers, investigators, and clinicians with recognized prominence in their respective fields.

SOURCES:

1. Bulletin of Information on National Board of Examinations, 1992. National Board of Medical Examiners.
2. Part III Examination General Instructions, Content Outlines and Sample Items, National Board of Medical Examiners, 1992.

Plans for Phased-In Implementation of Single Licensing Exam

The Federation of State Medical Boards (FSMB) and the National Board of Medical Examiners (NBME) have announced the signing of the agreement establishing the United States Medical Licensing Examination (USMLE), a single, uniform examination for medical licensure in the United States.

USMLE provides a common evaluation system to measure all applicants for medical licensure. The USMLE will replace the two currently existing examination sequences used in the medical licensing process: the FLEX and the certifying examinations of the NBME.

The USMLE is a progressive, three-step examination. All three steps must be completed to provide an adequate assessment for initial medical licensure. Step 1 focuses on key concepts of basic biomedical science with a special emphasis on principles and mechanisms underlying disease and modes of therapy. Step 2 focuses on clinical science considered essential for practice within a supervised setting. Step 3 will focus on aspects of biomedical and clinical science essential for the unsupervised practice of medicine.

Phase-in of the new examination began in 1992, with the first administration of the Step 1 examination in June 1992 and the first administration of Step 2 in September 1992. Current plans call for introduction of Step 3 in 1994. Phase-out of each current examination used for licensure will be complete by 1995. Further information regarding the phase-out was published in the March 1991 USMLE Special Bulletin and also is provided in the 1993 USMLE Bulletin of Information.

Key to Abbreviations

ACGME: Accreditation Council for Graduate Medical Education
AMA: American Medical Association
AOA: American Osteopathic Association
BPEAOA: Bureau of Professional Education of the American Osteopathic Association
CMA: Canadian Medical Association
CME: Council on Medical Education
ECFMG: Educational Commission for Foreign Medical Graduates (certificate)

continued

Key to Abbreviations–continued

FLEX: Federation Licensing Exam
FMG: Foreign Medical Graduate
FMGEMS: Foreign Medical Graduate Examination in the Medical Sciences
FSMB: Federation of State Medical Boards
IMG: International Medical Graduate
LCME: Liaison Committee for Medical Education (now replaced by the ACGME)
LMCC: Licentiate Medical Council of Canada (examination)
NBOME: National Board of Osteopathic Medical Examiners
NBME: National Board of Medical Examiners (examination)
NBOE: National Board of Osteopathic Examiners (examination)
PGY-1: Postgraduate year one
RCPSC: Royal College of Physicians and Surgeons of Canada
SPEX: Special Purpose Exam
USMG: U.S. Medical School Graduate
USMLE: U.S. Medical Licensing Examination
VQE: Visa Qualifying Exam

Alabama

For Information and Application

Cecile Waldrop
Director of Licensure
Board of Medical Examiners
P.O. Box 946
Montgomery, AL 36102
(205) 242-4116

TO TAKE FLEX (USMG)

All candidates must satisfy the following requirements:

1) Diploma showing graduation from a college of medicine or osteopathy.
2) One year of AMA- or AOA-approved internship or residency.
3) Two written character statements from two currently licensed physicians.
4) Complete necessary application forms.

TO TAKE FLEX (FMG)
Same requirements as for USMG with the addition of having an ECFMG certificate. Oral exam is required unless the applicant has been certified or recertified by an AMA Specialty Board within the past ten years.

Those who graduated from a nonapproved LCME school after February 11, 1988, must have their medical school approved by the Board of Medical Examiners.

Acceptable Licensing Exams
1) NBME.
2) FLEX (provided candidate was licensed in state in which FLEX was taken).
3) LMCC.
4) State exams prior to FLEX except Florida licensure exam.

To Receive State License
All candidates must satisfy the following requirements:
1) Pass acceptable licensing exam.
2) Take an oral exam given by the Board, except when applicant has passed a written licensing exam within ten years prior to application or has been certified or recertified by an AMA Specialty Board within ten years of application.
3) Licensure through a Fifth Pathway program is not acceptable.

Deadline for FLEX Application
March 1 for June exam: September 1 for December exam.

Registration and Exam Fees
Application Fee: $175.
FLEX Exam Fee: $420.
Oral Exam Fee: $400.

Alaska
For Information and Application
Nancy Ferguson
Licensing Examiner
Dept. of Commerce & Economic Development
State Medical Board
P.O. Box 110806
Juneau, AK 99811-0806
(907) 465-2541

TO TAKE FLEX (USMG)

All candidates must satisfy the following requirements:

1) Proof of an M.D. or D.O. degree.
2) Completed PGY-1 of AMA-approved internship or residency.
3) FLEX exam is given only to applicants who are applying for permanent licensure in Alaska.

TO TAKE FLEX (FMG)

Same requirements as for USMG with addition of having an ECFMG certificate.

Acceptable Licensing Exams

1) FLEX.
2) NBME.
3) The Board may consider state Board exams that are/were equivalent to FLEX; a complete breakdown of subjects and scores is required.

To Receive State License

All candidates must satisfy the following requirements:

1) Be a U.S. citizen or show proof of permanent resident status.
2) Pass FLEX, NBME, NBOME, or equivalent state exam.
3) Be personally interviewed by at least one member of the Board.
4) Licensure through a Fifth Pathway program is not acceptable.

Deadline for FLEX Application

120 days prior to the exam.

FLEX Registration and Exam Fees

Application: $50.
Examination: $500.
Reexamination: $500.
Initial License: $400.

Arizona (M.D.)

For Information and Application

Char McCall
Manager, Licensure Dept.
Board of Medical Examiners
2001 W. Camelback Rd.
Suite 300
Phoenix, AZ 85015
(602) 255-3751

TO TAKE FLEX (USMG)

All candidates must satisfy the following requirements:

1) Have a medical degree from a recognized and acceptable school of medicine.
2) Have completed one year of internship or residency in an ACGME-, AMA-, RCPSC-, or Association of American Colleges-approved U.S. or Canadian hospital program.
3) All applicants are subject to investigation, review, and examination, if deemed necessary by the Board. This also may include physical examination and/or mental evaluation.

TO TAKE FLEX (FMG)

All candidates must satisfy the following requirements for licensure, but may take FLEX after nine months of training during approved residency training:

1) Have an M.D. degree or its equivalent from a recognized and acceptable school of medicine.
2) Must have successfully completed a Fifth Pathway program and an additional 24 months of postgraduate medical education in an approved U.S. or Canadian hospital program and hold the standard ECFMG certificate that is valid indefinitely, or must have successfully completed 36 months of approved postgraduate medical education in an ACGME-, AMA-, RCPSC-, or Association of American Medical Colleges-approved U.S. or Canadian hospital program or have served as a full-time faculty member (Clinical Instructor, Assistant Professor, or higher) in an approved school of medicine in the United States or Canada for a total of 36 months.
3) Provide evidence of proficiency in the English language.
4) FMGs must fulfill clinical clerkship(s) training in the United States as part of the curriculum of a foreign school of medicine. This training must have been obtained either in a hospital affiliated with an approved school of medicine in the United States or an approved hospital residency program in the specialty area in which the clinical training is obtained.
5) All applicants are subject to investigation, review, and examination if deemed necessary by the Board. This also may include physical examination and/or mental evaluation.

Acceptable Licensing Exams

1) FLEX. Both components of FLEX must be passed within a three-year period.
2) NBME.
3) LMCC.
4) Complete written exam taken in one of these United States prior to the implementation of FLEX.
5) FLEX prior to 1985. Must receive a grade of 70 in each day and a FLEX weighted average of not less than 75. Must be achieved in one sitting.

To Receive State License

All candidates must have passed a complete written examination or one of the acceptable licensing exams. If the candidate's date of successful passage of a complete written exam was more than 10 years preceding the application, he must submit to a SPEX written examination.

Deadline for FLEX Application

March 1 for the June exam and September 1 for the December exam.

Deadline for SPEX Application

November 30 for March exam; March 1 for June exam; May 30 for September exam; August 23 for December exam.

Registration and Exam Fees

$550.
Endorsement: $450.
Endorsement with SPEX: $550.

Arizona (D.O.)

For Information and Application

Phyllis Lundy
Administrative Assistant
Board of Osteopathic Examiners in Medicine and Surgery
1830 West Colter, #104
Phoenix, AZ 85015
(602) 255-1747

To Take Exam

Arizona offers FLEX as the licensing exam. In order to qualify for examination, candidates must meet the following requirements:

1) Be a graduate of a school of osteopathic medicine.
2) Be of good moral character.

3) Have completed one year of internship—AOA- or AMA-approved.
4) Be a U.S. citizen or a resident alien.
5) Make application to Arizona Osteopathic Board for an osteopathic license in Arizona.

Acceptable Licensing Exams

1) FLEX.
2) NBOE.
3) Reciprocity with another state (via exam).

To Receive State License

Candidates must have passed FLEX or NBOE or be currently licensed in another state and be in good standing. The Board maintains reciprocity with all states.

Deadline for Exam

For the FLEX: February 24 for the June exam and August 24 for the December exam.

Registration and Exam Fees

FLEX is given through the auspices of the Arizona Board of Medical Examiners. Physicians are now required to pay $475.

Arkansas

For Information and Application

Peggy Pryor Cryer
Executive Secretary
Arkansas State Medical Board
2100 Riverfront Drive
Suite 200
Little Rock, AR 72202
(501) 324-9410
FAX: (501) 324-9413

TO TAKE FLEX (USMG)

All candidates must satisfy the following requirements:

1) Be a citizen of the United States; first papers accepted.
2) Be a graduate of an AMA-approved U.S. or Canadian medical school or a graduate of an AOA-approved osteopathic school.
3) Be of good moral standing, as well as in good standing with the medical societies of every state in which the candidate has resided.
4) Have completed an internship or residency in a CME-approved hospital.

TO TAKE FLEX (FMG)
Same requirements as for USMG with the addition of having an ECFMG certificate and having the ability to read, write, and speak English fluently. Must be a U.S. citizen or have filed Declaration of Intention to become one.

Acceptable Licensing Exams
1) FLEX.
2) NBME.
3) USMLE.
4) LMCC.
5) NBOE.
6) State exam prior to 1975.

To Receive State License
All candidates must have passed FLEX, NBME, or USMLE or be currently licensed by another state and in good standing. FMGs must appear before the Board.

Deadline for FLEX Application
70 days prior to the exam.

Registration and Exam Fees
Component 1: $250.
Component 2: $300.
Both: $450.
Annual: $50 for licensed physicians.

Pass/Fail Rates
109 took the June 1992 FLEX; 99 passed.

California (M.D.)
For Information and Application
Licensing Program
Medical Board of California
1426 Howe Avenue, Suite 54
Sacramento, CA 95825-3236
(916) 263-2449

TO TAKE FLEX (USMG)
All candidates must satisfy the following requirements:
1) Have original diploma from an LCME- or CCME-approved medical school.
2) Must meet minimum curriculum requirements for

medical and premedical education (latter must include physics, chemistry, and biology or zoology).

3) Supply all necessary supporting documents and fees.

TO TAKE FLEX (FMG)

Same requirements as for USMG. In addition, all applicants must provide certification by the ECFMG. Noncitizens must provide the Board with their original license to practice medicine, a Declaration of Intention to become a U.S. citizen, or a petition for naturalization.

Acceptable Written Licensing Exams

1) FLEX (see note below).
2) NBME.
3) Other written state Board exams (if taken and passed prior to June 1969).
4) Combination of NBME I/II and FLEX Component of two exams.
5) LMCC.
6) USMLE.
7) Combination of FLEX, USMLE, and NBME accepted by USMLE.

Note: Passing scores on the written exam will remain valid for purposes of qualifying to participate in postgraduate training or licensure in California for a period of 10 years from the month of examination, except that the validity may be extended by the Division for good cause and for time spent in a postgraduate training program, including, but not limited to, residency training, fellowship training, and remedial or refresher training.

To Receive State License

Pass approved written licensing exam as mentioned above, complete at least four months of postgraduate training in general medicine as part of the one-year postgraduate training requirement for licensure, and pass an oral examination. Those applicants who have practiced medicine for at least four years may be required to take additional exams.

Reciprocity Requirements

To be licensed by reciprocity, FMG candidates who have passed an acceptable written exam, have completed one year of ACGME/CCME-approved postgraduate training, and who have practiced medicine for at least four years in the United States must meet the minimum education requirements and pass both SPEX and oral examinations. USMG applicants also must meet the same minimum requirements and pass an oral exam.

Deadline for FLEX Application
90 days prior to exam; however, if workload permits, applications may be submitted at any time.

Registration and Exam Fees
Application and Fingerprint Fee: $423
FLEX: $520. Initial Licensing Fee: $500; however, a 50% reduction of this fee ($250) is allowed for applicants enrolled in an ACGME-approved postgraduate training program at the time of licensure.

California (D.O.)

For Information and Application

Osteopathic Medical Board of California
444 North Third Street
Suite A-200
Sacramento, CA 95814
(916) 322-4306

To Take Exam
All candidates must satisfy the following requirements:

1) Be a graduate of an AOA-approved school of osteopathic medicine.
2) Have completed one year of internship/residency with at least four months of medicine.

Acceptable Licensing Exams

1) NBOE.
2) Other acceptable written exams in osteopathic medicine.

To Receive State License
Candidates must pass a written exam as specified or approved by the Board that includes osteopathic principles and practices and also an oral/practical exam administered by the Board in which the applicant achieves a minimum grade of 75. Reciprocity is granted if the candidate holds an unrestricted license in osteopathic medicine in another state whose written licensing exam is recognized and approved by the Board (candidate still must pass the oral/practical exam of the California Board).

Deadline for Exam

30 days prior to the exam date. Exams are given at least twice each year.

Registration and Examination Fees

Original or Reciprocity License: $400, plus fingerprint fee.
Renewal-Active: $175/year.
Inactive: $150/year.

Colorado

For Information and Application

Board of Medical Examiners
1560 Broadway, Suite 1300
Denver, CO 80202
(303) 894-7690

TO TAKE FLEX (USMG)

All candidates must satisfy the following requirements:

1) Apply for licensure in Colorado.
2) Provide proof of medical school diploma to take Component 1.
3) Provide proof of candidate is in or has completed one year of postgraduate training to take Component 2.

TO TAKE FLEX (FMG)

All candidates must satisfy the following requirements:

1) Apply for licensure in Colorado.
2) Provide proof of passage of ECFMG exam.
3) Provide proof of medical school diploma to take Component 1.
4) Provide proof candidate is in second year or has completed two years of postgraduate training for Component 2.

Acceptable Licensing Exams

1) FLEX.
2) NBME.

To Receive State License

All candidates must have passed one of the acceptable licensing exams or, if licensed by state exam, must have a current unrestricted license in that state. USMGs must have completed one year of approved postgraduate medical training. As of November 30, 1988, FMGs must have completed three years of approved postgraduate medical training in the United States or Canada.

Deadline for FLEX Application
March 20 for the June exam; September 20 for the December exam.

Registration and Exam Fees
Components 1 and 2: $659
Component 1: $659
Component 2: $659
Application Fee (No Exam): $329.

Connecticut
For Information and Application
Joseph Gillen, Ph.D.
Section Chief
Medical Licensure
Division of Medical Quality Assurance
150 Washington Street
Hartford, CT 06106
(203) 566-1035

TO TAKE FLEX (USMG)
All applicants must satisfy the following requirements:

1) Have a medical degree from an approved medical or osteopathic school.
2) Medical graduates must have two years ACGME-approved residency training or its equivalent. Osteopathic graduates must have one year of AOA or ACGME-approved rotating internship or residency training.

TO TAKE FLEX (FMG)
Same requirements as for USMG with addition of holding current ECFMG certification or having completed an approved Fifth Pathway program.

Acceptable Licensing Exams

1) FLEX.
2) NBME.
3) LMCC.
4) State Board exams taken prior to 1979 and prior to the implementation of the FLEX in that state.
5) USMLE

To Receive State License
Candidates must have passed one of the acceptable licensing exams or an acceptable combination of examination segments. No oral examinations or interviews are required for licensure.

Deadline for FLEX Application
FLEX application, federation form, and fee are required approximately 10 weeks prior to exam. Applicants should contact the Board directly.

Registration and Examination Fees
$450 plus cost of exam booklets.

Pass/Fail Rates
38 took the June 1992 administration of the FLEX; 21 passed (includes partial retakes).

Delaware

For Information and Application

Rosemarie S. Vanderhoogt
Office Manager
Board of Medical Practice
O'Neill Bldg., P.O. Box 1401
Dover, DE 19903
(302) 739-4522

TO TAKE FLEX (USMG)
All applicants must satisfy the following requirements:

1) Have a diploma from a medical or osteopathic school.
2) Completed one year of internship in the United States.
3) An applicant is not eligible to take the exam if he has taken FLEX on three previous occasions (in or out of Delaware).

TO TAKE FLEX (FMG)
Same requirements as for USMG with addition of having an ECFMG certificate.

Acceptable Licensing Exams

1) FLEX.
2) NBME.
3) Pre-1973 state Board examination.

To Receive State License
FMGs must have three years' postgraduate training in the United States. Candidates must have passed FLEX or be licensed in

another state by FLEX or by the NBME exam. Each candidate will be interviewed by two members of the Board. It is left to the candidate to contact Board members for interviews.

Deadline for FLEX Application
60 days prior to the exam.

Registration and Examination Fees

Application: $10.
Licensure: $169.
Exam: $600
Renewal Fee (every two years): $169.

Pass/Fail Rates
8 took the December 1992 FLEX exam; 5 passed.

District of Columbia

For Information and Application

Keith T. Keemer
Contact Representative
District of Columbia
Board of Medicine
605 G Street, N.W.
Room LL202
Washington, DC 20001
(202) 727-5365

TO TAKE FLEX (USMG)
All applicants must satisfy the following requirements:

1) Be at least 18 years of age.
2) Must not have been convicted of a crime of moral turpitude that bears directly on the applicant's fitness to be licensed.
3) Graduate of an accredited medical school or osteopathic school.
4) Completed at least one year of postgraduate training in a program accredited by the ACGME. All U.S. graduates receiving their medical degrees after January 1, 1990, shall complete two years of ACGME postgraduate training before being eligible for licensure by any means.

TO TAKE FLEX (FMG)

1) Must comply with USMG requirements 1 and 2.
2) Must have a valid standard ECFMG certificate.

3) Must have completed at least three years of postgraduate training in a program accredited by the ACGME.
4) Must provide a detailed description of all clinical clerkships.

Acceptable Licensing Exams

1) FLEX.
2) NBME.
3) A state-constructed exam (if taken prior to June 30, 1979).

To Receive License

Candidates must have passed one of the acceptable licensing exams. FLEX taken prior to January 1985 must have been passed (taken in one sitting) with a FLEX weighted average of 75. One who fails either component after January 1985 is permitted two additional opportunities to take that component again without additional training. Failure of a component of FLEX three times requires that the candidate complete one additional year of postgraduate clinical training. Candidates may take FLEX no more than six times.

Deadline for FLEX Application

March 10 for the June exam; September 10 for the December exam.

Registration and Exam Fees

Application and Examination: $532. Individuals who wish to take the FLEX in the District of Columbia must also apply for a license to practice medicine in the District.

Application Fee for License by Waiver of Examination: $180.

Florida (M.D.)

For Information and Application

Dorothy J. Faircloth
Executive Director
Board of Medicine
130 North Monroe Street
Tallahassee, FL 32399-0750
(904) 488-0595

TO TAKE FLEX (USMG)

All candidates must satisfy the following requirements:

1) Must be 21 years of age.
2) Must have graduated from an accredited U.S. or Canadian medical school.

3) Must have completed one year of ACGME-accredited postgraduate training.

TO TAKE FLEX (FMG)

All candidates must satisfy the following requirements:

1) Must be 21 years of age.
2) Must have completed one year of ACGME-accredited postgraduate training.
3) Applicants must be graduates of a certified foreign medical school registered with the World Health Organization and be certified by the Dept. of Professional Regulation as having met the standards required to accredit medical schools in the United States or a comparable standard.
4) Demonstrated competency in English, if the language of instruction was other than English, through presentation of an ECFMG English proficiency certificate or by a satisfactory grade on the test of spoken English of the Educational Testing Service or a similar test approved by rule of the Board.

Requirements for Graduates of Noncertified Foreign Medical Schools

Same requirements as for FMG with the addition of the following:

1) Applicants whose clinical clerkships were completed prior to November 28, 1984, or who had begun their clinical clerkships but not completed such training prior to November 28, 1984 (provided such training took no longer than three years to complete), are subject to an individual evaluation determining the quality of the clinical clerkship. Graduates of schools not accredited by the ACGME (excluding accredited Canadian schools or certified foreign medical schools) must demonstrate that the core clerkship received in the United States as part of the medical school curriculum was obtained either in a hospital affiliated with an ACGME-accredited school and the affiliation included the core clerkship training for that school in the relevant subject area or in a hospital that had, at the time the clerkship training was obtained, an ACGME-accredited residency program in the specialty area and in which the clinical training was being obtained.
2) Hold an active, valid ECFMG certificate.

3) After October 1, 1992, the applicant shall have completed three years of accredited postgraduate training in one specialty area.

Acceptable Licensing Examinations

1) FLEX, within ten years immediately preceding the filing of an application for licensure in Florida.
2) NBME, within ten years immediately preceding the filing of an application for licensure in Florida.

To Receive State License

Candidate must pass FLEX or NBME within ten years immediately preceding the filing of an application for license. An oral interview and/or examination may be required. Florida does not offer licensure via reciprocity, only via examination or endorsement.

Deadline for FLEX Application

March 1 and September 1 for USMGs; February 15 and August 15 for FMGs.

Registration and Exam Fees

Endorsement Application Fee: $350.
Licensure by examination based on FLEX or NBME within last ten years—Application Fee: $100.
Exam: $100 Application Fee; $500 Exam Fee; Total: $600.

Florida (D.O.)

For Information and Application

Board of Osteopathic Medicine
1940 N. Monroe St.
Tallahassee, FL 32399-0757
(904) 922-6725

Acceptable Licensing Exams

1) NBOME.
2) Other state Board as described below.

To Receive State License

The Board has endorsement with any state if applicant has taken and passed an exam in another state that is similar to or more difficult than the exam given in Florida and that has an osteopathic component. Licensure may be granted if candidate is a graduate of an accredited college of osteopathy, has passed all three parts of the National Osteopathic Boards, and fulfills all other requirements for licensure. The Board does not accept FLEX.

Georgia

For Information and Application

Andrew Watry
Executive Director
Composite State Board of Medical Examiners
166 Pryor St., S.W.
Atlanta, GA 30303
(404) 656-3913

TO TAKE FLEX (USMG)

All candidates must satisfy the following requirements:

1) Be a graduate of a medical school approved by the Board.
2) Be of good moral character.
3) Be a resident of the United States for at least one year.
4) Have one year of Board-approved internship or residency.

TO TAKE FLEX (FMG)

All candidates must satisfy the following requirements:

1) Be of good moral character.
2) Be a resident of the United States for at least one year.
3) Have Board-approved internship or residency in the United States or Canada (Canadian medical graduates only). Candidates who graduated before July 1, 1985, must have one year; those who graduated after July 1, 1985, must have three years' internship.
4) Possess ECFMG certification.
5) Have a copy of transcript mailed from candidate's medical school (must be postmarked from the country of origin of the medical school).
6) For clerkship in the United States, the Board must receive documentation from approved teaching hospitals.

Acceptable Licensing Exams

1) FLEX.
2) NBME.
3) National Osteopathic Boards.

4) Other state Board examinations approved by the Board.
5) LMCC (Canadian medical graduates only).

To Receive State License
Candidates must have passed one of the acceptable licensing exams. FLEX combination scores are accepted for exams prior to January 1, 1978, only. In these cases, only scores from the latest exam dates will be used in the calculation of the overall score. FLEX taken prior to June 1985 must have been passed in one sitting. Candidates may be required to appear personally before the Board.

Deadline for FLEX Application
March 16 for the June exam; September 1 for the December exam (approximately 90 days before exam date).

Registration and Exam Fees
FLEX (includes licensure fee): $555.
By endorsement:
Application: $135.
Licensure: $165.

Guam

For Information and Application
Teofila P. Cruz, M.S.
Health Professional
Licensure Administrator
Guam Board of Medical Examiners
P.O. Box 2816
Agana, Guam 96910
(671) 734-4589

TO TAKE FLEX (USMG)
All candidates must satisfy the following requirements:
1) Be a graduate of an AMA-approved medical school.
2) One year's residence in Guam.

TO TAKE FLEX (FMG)
All candidates must satisfy the following requirements:
1) Be a graduate of a Guam Board of Medical Examiners-approved medical school.
2) One year's residence in Guam.

Acceptable Licensing Exams

1) FLEX (all foreign graduates). Both components of the FLEX must be passed in one sitting with a weighted average of at least 75%.
2) NBME or FLEX (U.S. graduates).
3) Specialty Board examination (provided candidate plans to restrict his practice in Guam to the specialty and provided it is a recognized specialty).

To Receive License

Candidates must complete an AMA-approved residency program within the United States, must have passed one of the acceptable licensing exams, must be Board-eligible or Board-certified, must have practiced medicine or been in a medical training program during the two years prior to applying for licensure to practice medicine in Guam, and must submit an outline of plans for practicing medicine in Guam. Candidates must be willing to complete a personal interview upon request. No reciprocity is granted.

Deadline for FLEX Application

20 days prior to the exam date.

Registration and Exam Fees

Application Fee: $100.
License Fee: $100.
FLEX Exam: $465.

Hawaii (M.D.)

For Information and Application

Executive Secretary
State of Hawaii
Professional & Vocational Licensing Division
Dept. of Commerce & Consumer Affairs
1010 Richards St.
P.O. Box 3469
Honolulu, HI 96801
(808) 586-2708

TO TAKE FLEX (USMG)

All candidates must satisfy the following requirements:

1) Be a graduate of an LCME-accredited medical school.
2) Have served at least one year of residency in an ACGME-accredited program.

TO TAKE FLEX (FMG)
Same requirements as for USMG with addition of having either a Fifth Pathway certificate or an ECFMG certificate and serving at least two years in a U.S. residency program accredited by the ACGME.

Acceptable Licensing Exams
1) FLEX.
2) NBME.

To Receive State License
Candidates must have passed one of the two acceptable licensing exams. A temporary license may be issued to those who work under the supervision of a physician who holds a regular license in Hawaii. These individuals must meet all other requirements and must agree to take FLEX within 18 months of issuance of temporary license. However, as of June 1992, candidates may request an additional six-month extension from the Board.

Deadline for FLEX Application
110 days prior to exam.

Registration and Examination Fees
All candidates must submit two separate payments as instructed below:
1) A postal money order made payable to the "Federation of State Medical Boards of the United States, Inc.":
   Components 1 and 2: $420.
   Component 1 only: $220.
   Component 2 only: $275.
2) A check or money order for $150 made payable to "Commerce and Consumer Affairs."

Please submit payments with application by the appropriate filing deadline and make sure that the *payment to the "Federation" is done by postal money order.* If a postal money order for the appropriate amount is not submitted, payment will be returned and the candidate will not be able to sit for the examination.

Pass/Fail Rates
8 took the June 1992 exam; 5 passed.

Hawaii (D.O.)

For Information and Application

Executive Secretary
Board of Osteopathic Examiners
Professional & Vocational Licensing Division
Dept. of Commerce & Consumer Affairs
1010 Richards St.
P.O. Box 3469
Honolulu, HI 96801
(808) 586-2708

TO TAKE FLEX (USMG)

All candidates must satisfy the following requirements:

1) Be a graduate of an AOA- or AMA-accredited osteopathic school.
2) Have served at least one year of internship in a hospital approved by the AOA or in a hospital approved by the AMA.

Acceptable Licensing Exams

1) FLEX.
2) NBOE.

To Receive State License

The Board will issue a license by three methods:

1) Endorsement of NBOME certificate.
2) Endorsement of FLEX.
3) Reciprocity.

No temporary license will be issued by the Board.

Deadline for FLEX Application

110 days prior to the examination.

Registration and Examination Fees

All candidates must submit two separate payments as instructed below:

1) A postal money order made payable to the "Federation of State Medical Boards of the United States, Inc.":
   Components 1 and 2: $420.
   Component 1 only: $220.
   Component 2 only: $275.
2) A check or money order for $150 made payable to "Commerce and Consumer Affairs."

Please submit payments with application by the appropriate filing date and make sure that the *payment to the "Federation" is done by postal money order.* If a postal money order for the appropriate amount is not submitted, payment will be returned and the candidate will be unable to sit for the examination.

Idaho

For Information and Application

Donald L. Deleski
Executive Director
Idaho State Board of Medicine
280 North 8th St., Suite 202
Statehouse
Boise, ID 83720
(208) 334-2822

To Take USMLE (USMG)

All candidates must satisfy the following requirements:

1) Have a degree from an accredited medical or osteopathic school in the United States or Canada.
2) Completed one year of internship in the United States or Canada.

To Take USMLE (FMG)

Same requirements as for USMG with the addition of possessing a diploma from a Board-approved medical school, ECFMG certification, and three years of approved postgraduate training in the United States or Canada.

Acceptable Licensing Exams

1) USMLE.
2) FLEX.
3) NBME.

To Receive State License

Applicants must have passed USMLE, must be diplomates of the National Board of Medical Examiners, or must hold current licenses received after examination in another state. No license will be issued without a personal interview. An additional examination may be required.

Deadline for FLEX Application

75 days prior to the exam.

Registration and Exam Fee

$245, plus cost of exam.
Endorsement: $300.

Illinois

For Information and Application

Pat Eubanks, Manager
Medical Unit
Dept. of Prof. Regulations
320 W. Washington St., 3rd Fl.
Springfield, IL 62786
(217) 782-0458

TO TAKE FLEX (USMG)

All candidates must satisfy the following requirements:

1) Graduate must have completed a six-year postsecondary course of study consisting of at least two years of liberal arts instruction, two academic years of study in the basic medical sciences, and two academic years of study in the clinical sciences; while enrolled in the medical college that conferred the degree, the core rotations of which must have been completed in clinical teaching facilities owned, operated, or formally affiliated with the medical college that conferred the degree, or under contract in teaching facilities owned, operated, or affiliated with another medical college that is officially recognized by the jurisdiction in which the medical school that conferred the degree is located; or graduated from a medical or osteopathic college accredited by the LCME, the Committee on Accreditation of Canadian Medical Schools in conjunction with the LCME, or the BPEAOA.
2) Have at least four months of internship/residency in an approved U.S. or Canadian hospital program.

TO TAKE FLEX (FMG)

Same requirements as for USMG with the addition of having ECFMG, VQE, or FMGEMS certification, and having at least four months of internship/residency in an approved U.S. or Canadian hospital program.

Acceptable Licensing Exams

1) FLEX.
2) NBME.

3) LMCC.
4) NBOE.

To Receive State License
Request for license will be considered if applicant has passed FLEX, LMCC, NBME, or NBOE. If passed in another state, candidate must make application for endorsement and completion of either 12 or 24 months of internship/residency.

Registration and Exam Fees
FLEX Component 1: $306.60 for the June 1993 exam.
FLEX Component 2: $363.25 for the June 1993 exam.
FLEX Components 1 & 2: $512.60 for the June 1993 exam.

Indiana

For Information and Application
Sherry East (for endorsement licensure)
Carol Verhonik (for FLEX)
Health Professions Bureau
402 West Washington
Room 041
Indianapolis, IN 46204
(317) 232-2960

TO TAKE FLEX (USMG)
All candidates must satisfy the following requirements:

1) Have an M.D. or D.O. degree from a Board-approved medical or osteopathic school.
2) Submit transcript of grades.
3) Be enrolled in an approved postgraduate training program in a U.S. or Canadian residency program.

Note: Candidates who have taken Component 1 or 2 since June 1985 may take either component only three times.

TO TAKE FLEX (FMG)
Same requirements as for USMG with addition of having an ECFMG certificate and having successfully completed two years of postgraduate training in a U.S. or Canadian hospital or institution.

Acceptable Licensing Exams

1) FLEX.
2) NBME.

3) State Board exams equal to Indiana criteria at the time the exams were taken.

To Receive State License

Candidates must have passed one of the acceptable licensing exams and/or be currently licensed in another state. If a candidate is not currently licensed and is a USMG, he must have passed applicable exams and completed one year of postgraduate training.

FMG for endorsement only:

1) Pass ECFMG.
2) Pass state Board exam or FLEX.
3) Have two years' approved postgraduate training.
4) Be currently licensed in another state.

USMG for endorsement only: Requirements are the same but ECFMG not required and only one year of postgraduate training needed for licensure.

Deadline for FLEX Application

March 15 for the June exam; September 10 for the December exam.

Registration and Exam Fees

Component 1: $295.
Component 2: $350.
Both: $495.
No additional fee for licensure.
Licensure by Endorsement of National Board Scores: $200.

Pass/Fail Rates

17 took the June 1992 FLEX exam; 13 passed.

Iowa

For Information and Application

Ann M. Martino, Ph.D.
Executive Director
Board of Medical Examiners
State Capitol Complex
Executive Hills West
1209 East Court Avenue
Des Moines, IA 50319
(515) 281-5171

TO TAKE FLEX (USMG)

All candidates must satisfy the following requirements:

1) Submit notarized photostatic copy of valid medical diploma.
2) Submit completed application.
3) Other requirements as directed by the Board.

TO TAKE FLEX (FMG)

Same requirements as for USMG with the addition of:

1) Submit notarized photostatic copy of evidence of completion of one year of approved postgraduate training in the United States or Canada or submit notarized photostatic copy of verifiable evidence of acceptance into an approved postgraduate program in the United States or Canada of at least one year in length.
2) Submit notarized photostatic copy of current ECFMG certificate or notarized photostatic copy of a certificate showing completion of an approved Fifth Pathway program.

Acceptable Licensing Exams

1) FLEX.
2) NBME.
3) NBOE.

To Receive State License

Candidates must comply with all licensing requirements and must pass FLEX, NBME, NBOE (osteopathic) or have a license to practice medicine and surgery that was issued by the duly constituted authority of another state, as a result of that state's written exam, if the state's exam is acceptable to the Iowa Board. Applicants must pass both Components 1 and 2 of FLEX with a score of 75 or better. Candidates who hold a Canadian license must submit proof of successful completion of exam administered by the LMCC. An oral interview may be required at the discretion of the Board.

Deadline for FLEX Application

March 15 for the June exam; September 15 for the December exam.

Registration and Exam Fees

Component 1 only: $300.
Component 2 only: $350.

Both: $500.

All endorsement permanent licenses are $300, whether passing FLEX in Iowa or another state.

Pass/Fail Rates

186 took the June 1992 FLEX; 155 passed.

Kansas

For Information and Application

State Board of Healing Arts
235 S. Topeka Blvd.
Topeka, KS 66603
(913) 296-7413

TO TAKE FLEX 1 (USMG & FMG)

All candidates must satisfy the following requirements:

1) Be a graduate of an approved medical or osteopathic school.
2) FMG-VQE or ECFMG required if from a foreign medical school.

TO TAKE FLEX 2 (USMG)

All candidates must satisfy the following requirements:

1) Be a graduate of an approved medical or osteopathic school.
2) Have completed one year of approved U.S. postgraduate medical training.
3) Must have passed FLEX 1.*

TO TAKE FLEX 2 (FMG)

All candidates must satisfy the following requirements:

1) Be a graduate of an approved medical or osteopathic school.
2) Have been awarded an ECFMG-VQE certificate.
3) Have completed three years of approved postgraduate training (must include one year of U.S. postgraduate training).
4) Foreign medical school attended must have been in existence for at least 15 years.
5) Must have passed FLEX 1.

*Note: Both FLEX 1 and FLEX 2 must be passed for candidate to receive license. FLEX 1 must be passed before FLEX 2 is taken, unless they are taken at the same sitting. If FLEX 2 is passed and FLEX 1 is failed, FLEX 1 must be retaken.

Acceptable Licensing Exams

1) FLEX.
2) NBME.
3) Pre-FLEX state exams.
4) USMLE

To Receive State License

Candidates must have passed FLEX with a 75 or above. FLEX taken prior to 1985 must have been passed in one sitting.

Deadline for FLEX Application

March 1 for the June exam and September 1 for the December exam.

Registration and Exam Fees

Component 1: $275.
Component 2: $345.
Both: $525.

Licensure is an additional $150 when both FLEX 1 and 2 are passed.

Pass/Fail Rates (December 1992 FLEX)

9 took both Components: 2 passed. 29 took Component 1 only; 9 passed.

Kentucky

For Information and Application

Licensing Coordinator
Kentucky Board of Medical Licensure
Hurstbourne Office Park
310 Whittington Parkway, #1B
Louisville, KY 40222
(502) 429-8046

TO TAKE FLEX (USMG)

All candidates must satisfy the following requirements:

1) Submit proof of graduation from a Board-approved medical school.
2) To take Component 1, candidate must be either currently enrolled in a postgraduate training program; or have completed a minimum of one year of postgraduate training in the United States approved by the ACGME; or enrolled in a postgraduate training program in Canada,

approved by the National Joint Committee of Preregistration Physician Training Programs; or will have completed this training within six months of taking this exam.

3) To take Component 2, candidate must have completed one year of postgraduate training in the United States approved by the ACGME; or a minimum of one year of postgraduate training in Canada approved by the National Joint Committee of Preregistration Physician Training Programs; or will have completed this training within six months of taking this exam.
4) To take Component 2, candidate must have passed FLEX Component 1, with a grade of 75 or better if applying only for Component 2.

TO TAKE FLEX (FMG)

All candidates must satisfy the following requirements:

1) Submit proof of graduation from a Board-approved medical school.
2) To take Component 1, candidate must be either currently enrolled in a postgraduate training program; or have completed a minimum of one year of postgraduate training in the United States approved by the ACGME; or enrolled in a postgraduate training program in Canada approved by the National Joint Committee of Preregistration Physician Training Programs; or will have completed this training within six months of taking this exam.
3) To take Components 1 and 2, candidate must possess a permanent ECFMG certificate.
4) To take Component 2, candidate must have completed a minimum of two years of postgraduate training in the United States approved by the ACGME; or a minimum of two years of postgraduate training in Canada approved by the National Joint Committee of Preregistration Physician Training Programs.
5) To take Component 2, candidate must have passed FLEX Component 1 with a grade of 75 or better if applying only for Component 2.

All applicants taking Components 1 and 2 in one sitting must meet the requirements for both Components 1 and 2. Should the applicant fail either part of FLEX (Components 1 or 2), he may retake that section only without having to repeat the section already passed. Applicants failing the FLEX, or any component thereof, three or more times previously in any state are not eligible to sit for the FLEX in Kentucky.

Acceptable Licensing Exams

1) FLEX.
2) State Boards.
3) NBME.
4) LMCC.
5) NBOE.

To Receive State License
USMGs need one year of approved postgraduate training: FMGs need three years. Candidates must have passed one of the acceptable licensing exams or hold a full and unrestricted medical license issued by a U.S. licensing Board or Canadian province as a result of passing a licensing exam with a grade of 75. The Board will accept a graduate of a Fifth Pathway program if the candidate passes the ECFMG exams.

Deadline for FLEX Application
March 1 for the June exam; September 1 for the December exam.

Registration and Exam Fees
Component 1: $250.
Component 2: $300.
Both (one sitting): $500.
Fees include the exam only; Kentucky licensure fee is additional. Passage of the FLEX in Kentucky does not lead to automatic licensure in the state. Applicants must apply and meet all requirements for licensure.

Pass/Fail Rates (June 1992 FLEX)
3 took both Components; 2 passed both, 1 failed Component 1 and passed Component 2.
3 took Component 1 only; 1 passed.

Louisiana

For Information and Application
Cheryl Neason (FLEX-USMG)
Melanie Walker (SPEX and reciprocity-USMG)
Merian Glasper (FMG exam and reciprocity)
Board of Medical Examiners

830 Union St., Suite 100
New Orleans, LA 70112
(504) 524-6763

TO TAKE FLEX (USMG)

All candidates must satisfy the following requirements:

1) Submit original medical diploma.
2) Submit completed application form, which includes two character references from physicians of immediate past location, providing candidate was there at least six months.
3) Be at least 21 years old and of good moral character.
4) If not a citizen, supply proof of legal entry or certificate of naturalization.

TO TAKE FLEX (FMG)

Same requirements as for USMG with the following additions:

1) Must have an ECFMG certificate.
2) Must demonstrate the ability to speak, understand, read, and write English.
3) Must present a valid visa issued by the United States, if the candidate is not a U.S. citizen.
4) Candidates must meet all requirements for full, unrestricted licensure; no temporary licenses will be issued.
5) Must have successfully completed three years of AMA-approved postgraduate training in a U.S. or Canadian program.

Acceptable Licensing Exams

1) FLEX.
2) NBME.
3) SPEX.

To Receive State License

Candidates must have passed FLEX in Louisiana or another state and must make a personal appearance before a member of the Board. No candidate will be considered for a license who has taken FLEX more than four times. Full licensure is required prior to beginning residency.

Note: If licensure was issued on the basis of a state exam, FLEX or NBME, and candidate has not had an exam within 10 years, SPEX must be taken. However, if candidate is certified (having taken an exam for an American Specialty Board approved by the AMA), straight reciprocity applies.

Deadline for FLEX Application
Two weeks after match-day announcement in June; second Friday in September.

Registration and Exam Fees
$520.
Reciprocity: $200.
Reciprocity and SPEX: $475.

Maine (M.D.)
For Information and Application
David R. Hedrick
Executive Director
Board of Registration in Medicine
State House Station, #137
Augusta, ME 04333
(207) 287-3601

TO TAKE FLEX (USMG)
All candidates must satisfy the following requirements:

1) Must be a graduate of an accredited medical school in the United States or Canada.
2) Must be of good moral character.
3) If graduated after January 1, 1970, must have completed at least 24 months in an approved U.S. or Canadian internship/residency program.
4) If graduated before January 1, 1970, must have completed at least 12 months in an approved U.S. or Canadian internship/residency program. (Board may find postgraduate training taken in other countries to be equivalent.)

TO TAKE FLEX (FMG)
Same requirements as for USMG with the following differences:

1) Must have completed 36 months in an approved U.S. or Canadian internship/residency program. (Board may find postgraduate training taken in other countries to be equivalent.)

2) Have taken FMGEMS or VQE exams and hold ECFMG certification.

Acceptable Licensing Exams

1) FLEX.
2) NBME.
3) LMCC.
4) USMLE.
5) State Board exam equivalent to any of the previously mentioned exams.
6) During USMLE phase-in, individual components of FLEX, NBME, or USMLE may be combined to give credit for passage of licensing exam requirement. Inquire with Board.

To Receive State License

Candidates must have passed one of the acceptable licensing exams and must submit to an oral exam administered by the Maine Board. Each component of the FLEX exam must be passed. Application for endorsement of a license from another state must be filed at least 60 days prior to relocation in Maine.

Deadline for FLEX Application

75 days prior to test date.

Registration and Exam Fees

FLEX: $420.
Application Fee: $300.
Oral Exam Fee: $50.
Licensure by endorsement of NBME or other state licensing exam: $350 ($300 application fee, plus $50 oral exam fee).

Maine (D.O.)

For Information and Application

Susan E. Strout
Executive Secretary
Board of Osteopathic Exam & Registration
State House Station #142
Augusta, ME 04333
(207) 287-2480

Acceptable Licensing Exams

1) FLEX.
2) NBOE.
3) State Board equivalent to NBOE exam.

To Receive State License

Candidates must have graduated from an accredited school of osteopathic medicine, successfully completed one year of rotating internship in an AOA-approved institution or another postgraduate program deemed equivalent by the Board, and passed one of the licensing exams noted above.

Registration and Exam Fees

Endorsement of Licensure: $400 biennially.
FLEX: $490.

Maryland

For Information and Application

J. Michael Compton
Executive Director
Board of Physician Quality Assurance
P.O. Box 2571
Baltimore, MD 21215-0095
(410) 764-4777

Acceptable Licensing Exams

1) FLEX.
2) NBME.
3) NBOE (for D.O. who passed exam after January 1, 1971).
4) State medical Board exam accepted if in compliance with Maryland statutory requirements.

Deadline for FLEX Application

March 1 for the June exam and September 1 for the December exam.

Exam Fees

Component 1: $415.
Component 2: $505.
Both: $770.

Massachusetts

For Information and Application

Licensing Clerk
Board of Registration in Medicine
Ten West Street
Boston, MA 02111
(617) 727-3086

Note: Indicate whether USMG or FMG.

Requests for Applications (FLEX Exams):
LGR Examinations
Attn: MA FLEX Program
1315 South Allen Street
State College, PA 16801-5992
1-800-877-3926

TO TAKE FLEX (USMG)
The following is a partial list of the Board's requirements; a full list will be sent with the candidate's application form. Candidate must:

1) Possess a medical school diploma and complete the application form.
2) No postgraduate training in the United States required for Component 1.
3) To sit for Component 2, candidate must have one year of postgraduate training in the United States in an ACGME-approved program.

TO TAKE FLEX (FMG)
Same requirements as for USMG with addition of having a valid ECFMG certificate. Direct verification of medical education is required. All information must be received 90 days prior to the exam. Candidate should enclose a self-addressed, postage-paid envelope when requesting an application. A complete list of the Board's requirements will be sent with the application. Contact LGR Examinations to request applications for FLEX exam.

Acceptable Licensing Exams

1) FLEX.
2) NBME.
3) NBOE.
4) LMCC (for graduates of Canadian schools only) and a current provincial license.
5) Any state Board exam taken before 1970.
6) Will license on the basis of the American Specialty Board exam if none of the above exams taken.

To Receive State License
Contact the Board for full information. Send a 9″ x 12″ envelope (98¢ postage for USMGs and $1.44 postage for FMGs).

1) State whether you are a graduate of a U.S. medical school or a foreign medical school. (FMG)
2) A 75 weighted average is required if FLEX exam was taken prior to 1985. Split FLEX is not accepted; exam must be passed in one sitting. A minimum score of 75 is required for Components 1 and 2 of the current FLEX exam.
3) Enclose curriculum vitae.
4) USMG: For full licensure, 1 year of ACGME-approved training. FMG: 2 years of ACGME (US) required.

Registration and Exam Fees

Fees subject to change.
Limited License: $50 per year.
Temporary License: $175.
Lapsed License: $375.
Full License: $350.
Renewals: $250 every two years on applicant's birthday.*
Exam Fees: Component 1: $307.
Component 2: $352.
Components 1 and 2: $570.

*Renewal of your license will be required on your first birthday after the license issuance date. Once the license is renewed on your birthday, it will then be valid for a full two-year period. The only exception to the above requirement would be if your first birthday falls within 90 days of obtaining initial licensure. If your first birthday falls within this time frame, you will not be required to renew until the following birthday.

Michigan (M.D.)

For Information and Application

Board of Medicine
P.O. Box 30192
Lansing, MI 48909
(517) 373-9102

TO TAKE FLEX (USMG)

All candidates must satisfy the following requirements:

1) Must be a graduate of a medical school approved by the Board.
2) Must complete six months of postgraduate training in a program approved by the Board in a Board-approved hospital or institution to sit for FLEX 2.

TO TAKE FLEX (FMG)

1) Must have passed the examination developed and administered by ECFMG.
2) Must complete six months of postgraduate training in a program approved by the Board in a Board-approved hospital or institution to sit for FLEX 2.

Acceptable Licensing Exams

1) FLEX.
2) NBME.

To Receive License (USMG)

1) Must have graduated from an LCME-accredited school.
2) Must pass an exam approved by the Board.
3) Must complete two years of postgraduate training in a program approved by the Board in a Board-approved hospital or institution.

To Receive License (FMG)

1) Must complete the requirements for a degree in medicine as defined by rule.*
2) Must pass an exam approved by the Board.
3) Must have passed examination developed and administered by the ECFMG.
4) Must complete three years of postgraduate training in a program approved by the Board in a Board-approved hospital or institution; two years if candidate has passed VQE, FMGEMS, or Part I and Part II of NBME.

**Rule: Complete the requirements for a degree in medicine means the satisfactory completion of a medical educational program covering a period of at least 130 weeks, devoted to a course of study in the basic science curriculum that includes, at minimum, anatomy, biochemistry, microbiology, physiology, pharmacology, preventive medicine and pathology, and clinical clerkships in at least surgery, obstetrics and gynecology, psychiatry, pediatrics, and internal medicine. All clerkships shall be completed in a hospital or institution located in the United States or Canada and approved by the Board or a hospital or institution that offers a postgraduate clinical training program in the content area of the clerkship.*

Deadline for FLEX Application

90 days before the next scheduled examination.

Registration and Exam Fees

Licensure by examination: $90.

Licensure by endorsement (must have current, active license in another state): $90.

Michigan Controlled Substance License: $60.

FLEX Component 1: $289.

FLEX Component 2: $344.

FLEX Components 1 and 2: $544.

There is a $50 nonrefundable application fee for FLEX exams. Call 1-800-847-7171 for an application.

Michigan (D.O.)

For Information and Application

Board of Osteopathic Medicine & Surgery
Dept. of Licensing & Regulation
P.O. Box 30018
Lansing, MI 48909
(517) 373-9102

To Take Exam

All candidates must satisfy the following requirements:

1) Be a graduate of an AOA-approved school of osteopathic medicine.
2) Have commenced training in a one-year AOA-approved hospital internship program prior to taking the exam.

Acceptable Licensing Exams

1) NBOE.
2) Michigan does not administer the FLEX to its osteopathic physicians and surgeons.

To Receive State License

Candidates must have passed one of the acceptable licensing exams. One-year training requirement must be completed before license is granted. The Board may accept endorsement of another state's license if the standards of the state granting the license are substantially equivalent to Michigan's for the year the candidate was licensed.

Deadline for Exam Application

March 15 for the April exam; September 15 for the October exam.

Registration and Exam Fees

D.O. Application Without Exam: $90.

(For licensure by endorsement, applicant must have current active license in another state.)

Minnesota

For Information and Application

Executive Director
Board of Medical Practice
2700 University Ave., West
Suite 106
St. Paul, MN 55114-1080
(612) 642-0538

TO TAKE FLEX (USMG)

All applicants must satisfy the following requirements:

1) Submit certified copy of medical or osteopathic diploma received from recognized school.
2) Submit evidence of satisfactory application and acceptance into an approved residency.
3) Submit one notarized personal photograph.
4) Have a personal interview before the Board.

Note: U.S. or Canadian medical school graduates are allowed to take FLEX during the final quarter of their senior year of medical school if they can show evidence of their standing. They also must show evidence of acceptance into an approved residency program.

TO TAKE FLEX (IMG)

Same requirements as for USMG with addition of having an ECFMG certificate. Applicants must show evidence of acceptance into an approved internship program. Fifth Pathway candidates may be accepted. Originals of all basic documents must be presented at the interview.

Acceptable Licensing Exams

1) FLEX.
2) NBME.
3) NBOE.
4) LMCC.

To Receive State License

Candidates must have submitted all required fees and credentials and must have passed with a 75 score on one of the acceptable licensing exams. IMGs must have completed two years of approved U.S./Canadian postgraduate training.

Deadline for FLEX Application
March 1 for the June exam; September 1 for the December exam.

Registration and Exam Fees
Application: $200.
Exam: $490.
Annual: $168.

Mississippi

For Information and Application
Frank J. Morgan, Jr., M.D.
Executive Officer
Board of Medical Licensure
2688-D Insurance Center Drive
Jackson, MS 39216
(601) 354-6645

TO TAKE FLEX (USMG)
All candidates must satisfy the following requirements:

1) Must present M.D. from an LCME-accredited school of medicine or D.O. from an AOA-accredited school of osteopathic medicine.
2) Must be at least 21 years of age and of good moral character.
3) Must make personal appearance before the Board.

TO TAKE FLEX (FMG)
All candidates must satisfy the following requirements:

1) Must be at least 21 years of age and of good moral character.
2) Must present medical degree from a reputable medical college.
3) Must have ECFMG, VQE, or FMGEMS certification.
4) Must have completed at least three years of postgraduate training in the United States or Canada accredited by the ACGME or RCPSC.
5) Must make a personal appearance before the Board.
6) Candidates applying through a Fifth Pathway program must meet the same requirements previously mentioned.

Each Fifth Pathway candidate is considered on an individual basis.

Acceptable Licensing Exams

1) FLEX.
2) NBME.
3) LMCC.
4) NBOE.
5) Licensing exams given by most states prior to March 8, 1973.

To Receive State License

Candidates must have passed FLEX or hold a current license received via FLEX in another state and must have met all other licensure requirements. A personal interview with the Executive Officer of the Board is required.

Deadline for FLEX Application

March 24 for the June exam; September 23 for the December exam.

Registration and Exam Fees

Component 1 only: $325.
Component 2 only: $375.
Both: $500.

Missouri

For Information and Application

Tina Steinman
State Board of Registration for the Healing Arts
P.O. Box 4
Jefferson City, MO 65102
(314) 751-0098

TO TAKE FLEX (USMG)

All candidates must satisfy the following requirements:

1) Be a graduate of a medical or osteopathic school approved by the Board.
2) Complete one year of AMA-/AOA-approved postgraduate training.
3) Supply all necessary supporting documents.

TO TAKE FLEX (FMG)

Same requirements as for USMG with addition of having a permanent, valid indefinitely ECFMG certificate. Must provide proof of eligibility of licensure in country of graduation. Graduates from medical schools located in Mexico may complete a Fifth Pathway program in lieu of proof of eligibility of licensure in country of graduation. Must have completed three years of AMA-approved training in one recognized specialty in the United States.

Acceptable Licensing Exams

1) FLEX.
2) NBME.
3) Written state Board exams that include basic science subjects.

To Receive State License
Candidates must have passed FLEX or hold a license in another state that was obtained via a written exam noted in #3 of the preceding section. FMGs must have completed three years of AMA-approved training in the United States. Missouri statute does not provide for licensure by direct reciprocity with the LMCC.

Deadline for FLEX Application
April 1 for the June exam; October 1 for the December exam.

Registration and Exam Fees
Component 1 only: $250.
Component 2 only: $300.
Both: $450.

Pass/Fail Rates (December 1992 FLEX)
13 took both Components: 12 passed: 2 took Component 2 only; 2 passed.

Montana

For Information and Application
Carol Berger Norling
Administrative Assistant
Board of Medical Examiners
Department of Commerce
111 N. Jackson
Helena, MT 59620
(406) 444-4284 or 444-4276

TO TAKE FLEX (USMG)
All candidates must satisfy the following requirements:

1) Be a graduate of a Board-approved medical or osteopathic school for Component 1.

2) Completed one year of AMA- or AOA-approved postgraduate training for Component 2.
3) Application must be certified by the medical school; applicant must submit copy of diploma and internship certificate, plus two pictures of himself.

TO TAKE FLEX (FMG)

Same requirements as for USMG with addition of having an ECFMG, VQE, FMGEMS, or Fifth Pathway program certificate (for U.S. citizens only).

Acceptable Licensing Exams

1) FLEX.
2) NBME.
3) NBOE.
4) LMCC.
4) Other state licensing exams except Florida's.

To Receive State License

1) Candidates must have passed one of the acceptable licensing exams or currently hold a valid license in another state that was obtained by passing a written exam in that state. FLEX may not have been taken more than three times in any state.
2) FMGs must have completed three years of postgraduate training in an AMA-approved institution.
3) FMGs may make a personal appearance before the Board.

Deadline for FLEX Application

March 15 for the June exam; September 5 for the December exam.

Registration and Exam Fees

Component 1: $270.
Component 2: $325.
Both: $520.

Pass/Fail Rates (June 1992 FLEX)

Rates not available.

Nebraska

For Information and Application

Katherine A. Brown
Executive Secretary

Board of Examiners in Medicine and Surgery
P.O. Box 95007
Lincoln, NE 68509
(402) 471-2115

TO TAKE FLEX (USMG)
All candidates must submit a certified copy of their medical diploma.

TO TAKE FLEX (FMG)
Same requirements as for USMG with addition of having a permanent, valid indefinitely ECFMG certificate. Proof of graduation from foreign medical schools whose graduates participate in Fifth Pathway programs, together with the completion of a one-year Fifth Pathway program, is considered to be equivalent to receiving a U.S. medical degree.

Acceptable Licensing Exams
1) FLEX.
2) NBME.
3) LMCC.

To Receive State License
Candidates must have passed one of the acceptable licensing exams in Nebraska or in another state and have completed one year (USMG) or three years (FMG) of approved postgraduate training. Licenses via endorsement are issued to those candidates who possess medical licenses in any of the 50 states, or any of the U.S. territories, on an individual basis, provided the candidates have met the equivalent requirements to those that are statutory in Nebraska.

Deadline for FLEX Application
April 1 for the June exam; September 18 for the December exam.

Registration and Exam Fees
Exam: $476.
Reciprocity/Endorsement: $201.
Includes first license; renewals are $102, every two years.

Nevada (M.D.)
For Information and Application
Patricia R. Perry
Executive Director

Board of Medical Examiners
P.O. Box 7238
Reno, NV 89510
(702) 688-2559

TO TAKE FLEX (U.S./Canadian Graduates)

All candidates must satisfy the following requirements:

Component 1:

1) Candidate must have graduated from an approved medical school, having attended two years or more prior to graduation.
2) Candidate must not have failed any portion of FLEX more than two times.

Component 2:

1) Candidate must have graduated from an approved medical school, having attended two years or more prior to graduation.
2) Candidate must have successfully completed one year of graduate residency training in the United States or Canada approved by the ACGME or CCME.
3) Candidate must have successfully passed Component 1 of FLEX if only applying to sit for Component 2.
4) Candidate may not have failed any portion of FLEX more than two times.

TO TAKE FLEX (FMG)

Same requirements as for U.S. Canadian graduates, with the addition of having passed ECFMG or FMGEMS. Prior to taking FLEX in Nevada, candidate must furnish the Board with verification of ECFMG certification.

Reexaminations

1) If an applicant fails the examination required for licensing, whether taken in Nevada or elsewhere, he may be reexamined after not less than six months.
2) If he fails the examination on his second attempt, he is not entitled to a third attempt within less than one year after the date of the second attempt. Before taking the examination for the third time, he shall furnish proof satisfactory to the Board of one additional year of training as a resident, completed after his second attempt to pass the examination.

3) If an applicant fails the examination after three attempts, he must show the Board by clear and convincing evidence that extraordinary circumstances justify his taking the examination again.

Acceptable Licensing Exams

1) FLEX.
2) NBME.
3) State written exam with Board certification by the American Board of Medical Specialties.

To Receive State License

Candidates must have completed three years of postgraduate education in the United States or Canada (waiver possible for medically underserved areas) and must have successfully passed one of the acceptable licensing exams. An oral examination that covers basic medical competency is required, as well as a written, open-book examination of the state's medical practice act. The SPEX must be taken if it is more than ten years since the date of application for a license to practice medicine in this state. The applicant must have passed:

1) Part III of the examination given by the National Board of Medical Examiners.
2) Component II of the FLEX.
3) The examination for certification by a specialty Board of the American Board of Medical Specialties, and received certification by it.
4) SPEX.

For any examination conducted by the Board for a license to practice medicine, an applicant must answer correctly at least 75% of the questions propounded.

Deadline for FLEX Application

Applications for the exam must be on file 12 weeks before the exam, given in June and December.

Registration and Exam Fees

FLEX (Components 1 & 2)
Administration Fee: $200.
Examination Fee: $420.
Total: $620.
Component 1 Administration Fee: $100.
Examination Fee: $220.

Total: $320.
Component 2 Administration Fee: $100.
Examination Fee: $275.
Total: $375.

Nevada (D.O.)

For Information and Application

Larry J. Tarno, D.O.
Executive Director
Board of Osteopathic Medicine
2121 E. Flamingo
Las Vegas, NV 89119
(702) 732-2147

Acceptable Licensing Exams

NBOE, FLEX (FLEX exams can be arranged through the Nevada State Board of Medical Examiners).

To Receive State License

1) Candidate must have D.O. degree from college requiring actual attendance of 36 months and offering courses specified in the statute.
2) One year of internship in program conforming to AOA's minimum standards or three years of postgraduate training approved by the AMA and AOA.
3) Reciprocity is granted at the discretion of the Board.

Reregistration

Annual, January 1, Fee $100. 35 hours of CME required per year.

Application for License

Fee: $200.

New Hampshire

For Information and Application

Bd. of Registration in Medicine
2 Industrial Park Drive
Concord, NH 03301
(603) 271-1203

TO TAKE FLEX (USMG)

All candidates must satisfy the following requirements:

1) Be a graduate of a CME-accredited medical school.
2) Have completed satisfactorily two years of work in college or its equivalent.

3) Have completed two years of formal postgraduate training.
4) Submit letters of reference as required.
5) Have proof of commitment to practice in New Hampshire.
6) Fulfill other requirements designated by the Board, including a personal interview before a Board member.

Note: New Hampshire has not offered FLEX for several years and may not in the foreseeable future because of commitment requirement.

TO TAKE FLEX (FMG)
Same requirements as for USMG with addition of having an ECFMG certificate and making a personal appearance before the entire Board.

Acceptable Licensing Exams
1) FLEX.
2) NBME.
3) Another written state exam (at the discretion of the Board).

To Receive State License
A candidate must have satisfactorily passed one of the acceptable licensing exams. Licensure via endorsement is granted on an individual basis according to background and training. A permanent or temporary license is granted once all requirements are met.

New Jersey
For Information and Application
Charles A. Janousek
Executive Director
Board of Medical Examiners
28 West State St., Room 602
Trenton, NJ 08608
(609) 292-4843

TO TAKE FLEX (USMG)
All candidates must satisfy the following requirements:
1) Have graduated from a medical school accredited by LCME or AOA.
2) Have completed one year of approved postgraduate training.

TO TAKE FLEX (FMG)
Same requirements as for USMG. Passing score on ECFMG certification required for FMGs to take the New Jersey FLEX examination. A year of fellowship is not acceptable.

Acceptable Licensing Exams
1) FLEX.
2) NBME.
3) Another written state exam prior to December 31, 1972.

To Receive State License
Candidates must have passed one of the acceptable licensing exams. A CV or resume must be included with license application. No oral examination is required, but a personal interview may be necessary.

Deadline for FLEX Application
March 15 for the June exam; September 15 for the December exam.

Registration and Examination Fees
FLEX: $500
Biennial Registration Fee: $220.
Licensure Fee by Endorsement: $225.

New Mexico (M.D.)
For Information and Application
Board of Medical Examiners
491 Old Santa Fe Trail
Lamy Bldg. 2nd Floor
P.O. Box 20001
Santa Fe, NM 87504
(505) 827-9933

TO TAKE FLEX (USMG)
All candidates must satisfy the following requirements:
1) Be of good moral character.
2) Have graduated from an approved U.S. or Canadian medical school.
3) Have completed one year of postgraduate training in an approved U.S. or Canadian hospital program.
4) Completed application for licensure, including an interview before the secretary-treasurer of the Board.
5) Submitted medical school transcripts.

TO TAKE FLEX (FMG)
Same requirements as for USMG with addition of having an ECFMG certificate and having a medical school diploma from an approved medical school. Two years of postgraduate training in an approved U.S. or Canadian hospital program are required. Copy of English translations of transcripts is necessary.

Acceptable Licensing Exams
1) FLEX.
2) NBME.
3) LMCC.

To Receive State License
Candidates must have passed FLEX or NBME. Two personal appearances, an interview with a Board member and one before the entire Board, are necessary for a permanent license. To receive license by endorsement, candidate must have passed an approved exam and have completed one year of postgraduate education. FMGs must have two years of postgraduate education in an approved U.S. or Canadian hospital program.

Note: The medical practice act is currently being updated in the 1993 New Mexico legislative session and may require two years of postgraduate education for everyone who applies for licensure.

Deadline for FLEX Application
Ten weeks prior to the exam.

Registration and Exam Fees
FLEX: $470.
Application: $350.
Triennial Renewal Fee: $210.

New Mexico (D.O.)

For Information and Application
Michelle McGinnis
Executive Director
New Mexico Board of Osteopathic Medical Examiners
P.O. Box 25101
Santa Fe, NM 87504
(505) 827-7171

Note: New Mexico offers the FLEX exam for osteopaths. The Board will accept a passing grade on FLEX or National Osteopathic Boards.

Acceptable Licensing Exams

1) FLEX.
2) NBOE.
3) Another written state examination.

To Receive State License

The Board will endorse FLEX, NBOE, or any state examination with requirements equal to New Mexico. One year AOA internship or AMA-approved postgraduate training is required. An oral interview is required.

Deadline for FLEX Application

10 weeks prior to exam.

Registration and Exam Fees

FLEX: (Combined): $500.
Licensure Fee: $300.
Renewal Fee: $100.

New York

For Information and Application

Thomas J. Monahan
Executive Secretary
N.Y. State Education Dept.
State Board for Medicine
Cultural Education Center
Room 3023
Empire State Plaza
Albany, NY 12230
(518) 474-3841

TO TAKE FLEX (USMG)

All candidates must satisfy the following requirements:

1) Must have completed two years acceptable preprofessional education.
2) Have graduated from an accredited U.S. or Canadian medical school.

TO TAKE FLEX (FMG)

All candidates must satisfy the following requirements:

1) Must have completed two years acceptable preprofessional education.
2) Must complete curriculum in medical school recognized as an acceptable educational program for physicians of

the country in which school is located and have received the degree of Doctor of Medicine or Doctor of Osteopathy or equivalent.

3) Must have passed a satisfactory proficiency examination. An applicant seeking licensure under a Fifth Pathway program must have been a U.S. resident prior to enrolling in a foreign medical school, must have completed all the requirements of that school, must have attained a satisfactory score on a qualifying exam, and must have completed one year of clinical clerkship.

To Be Eligible for Licensure (USMG)
All candidates must satisfy the above requirements (USMG) and:

1) Be a U.S. citizen or an alien lawfully admitted for permanent U.S. residence.
2) Have passed an acceptable licensing exam.
3) Have completed one year of acceptable postgraduate training.

To Be Eligible for Licensure (FMG)
All candidates must satisfy the above requirements (FMG) and:

1) Be a U.S. citizen or an alien lawfully admitted for permanent U.S. residence.
2) Have passed an acceptable licensing exam.
3) Have three years of ACGME- or AOA-approved postgraduate training.

Acceptable Licensing Exams

1) FLEX.
2) NBME.
3) NBOE.

To Receive State License
All applicants must meet the requirements specified above.

Deadline for FLEX Application
90 days prior to the exam.

Registration and Exam Fees

Biennial Registration Fee: $330.
Examination Fee: $260.
Total: $590.

North Carolina

For Information and Application

Bryant D. Paris, Jr.
Executive Secretary
Board of Medical Examiners
1203 Front Street
Raleigh, NC 27609
(919) 828-1212

TO TAKE FLEX (USMG)
All candidates should contact the Board six months prior to moving to North Carolina and must possess an approved medical school diploma.

TO TAKE FLEX (FMG)
All candidates must have an approved medical school diploma and must have an ECFMG certificate. Candidates must complete three years of postgraduate training to take the exam, unless they are enrolled in a training program in North Carolina.

Acceptable Licensing Exams

1) FLEX.
2) NBME.
3) Written state Board exams given prior to FLEX.
4) NBOE all parts taken after January 1, 1990.

To Receive State License
Candidates must have passed one of the acceptable licensing exams, must have completed one year of postgraduate training (three years of FMGs), must have appeared before the Board or the Executive Secretary for a credential review, and must have submitted the appropriate certificates and fees.

Deadline for FLEX Application
75 days prior to the exam.

Registration and Exam Fees

Component 1: $470.
Component 2: $525.
Components 1 and 2: $670.
Biennial Registration: $100.

North Dakota

For Information and Application

Lynette Lewis
Administrative Assistant
Board of Medical Examiners
City Center Plaza, Suite 12
418 E. Broadway Avenue
Bismarck, ND 58501
(701) 223-9485

Note: As of December 1986, the FLEX is no longer administered in North Dakota.

Acceptable Licensing Exams

1) FLEX.
2) NBME.
3) LMCC.

To Receive State License

Candidates must have passed one of the acceptable licensing exams (reciprocity is granted to a state medical license holder whose license was obtained via FLEX or a written state Board examination). We also endorse NBME or LMCC. Each physician must also meet our licensure requirements regarding residency training. An oral interview before the Board (in March, July, or November) is required.

Ohio

For Information and Application

Penny McKenzie
Chief of Licensure
State Medical Board
77 S. High St., 17th Floor
Columbus, OH 43266-0315
(614) 466-3934

TO TAKE FLEX (LCME or AOA-accredited medical school)

All candidates must satisfy the following requirements:

1) Must hold a diploma from a medical or osteopathic school in the United States or Canada.
2) Must have completed two years of undergraduate collegiate work or its equivalent.
3) Must have completed 12 months of approved internship,

residency, or clinical fellowship in the United States or Canada.

TO TAKE FLEX (medical school not accredited by LCME or AOA)
All candidates must satisfy the following requirements:

1) Must have two years of undergraduate collegiate work or its equivalent.
2) Must hold a valid ECFMG certificate unless they have completed a Fifth Pathway program.
3) Must have successfully completed no less than 12 months of approved internship, residency, or clinical fellowship in the United States or Canada, or the equivalent as determined by the Board. Those who pass the FLEX and who did not complete a Fifth Pathway program must submit satisfactory evidence to the Board of successful completion of not less than 24 months of approved postgraduate training through the second-year level of training to be eligible for licensure. A second application will be required at that time for licensure.
4) Must have achieved at least 230 on the Test of Spoken English (TSE) of the Educational Testing Service regardless of citizenship or country of birth unless:
   a) They have completed two years of undergraduate college work in the United States; or
   b) They have, during the five years immediately preceding the date of application, held an unrestricted license in another state and actively practiced medicine in the United States during that time; or
   c) They have completed a Fifth Pathway program.

Those who obtain a score of at least 210 but less than 230 on the TSE may petition the Board to make an appearance for purposes of demonstrating their ability to communicate adequately in spoken English.

Acceptable Licensing Exams

1) FLEX.
2) NBME.
3) LMCC.
4) Written state Board exams (subject to approval of the Ohio State Medical Board).

To Receive State License

Candidates must have passed FLEX, LMCC, or be a diplomate of the NBME/NBOME. Endorsement can be achieved if candidate holds a valid license from another state (subject to approval of the Ohio State Medical Board).

Deadline for FLEX Application

13 weeks prior to the exam.

Registration and Exam Fee

FLEX: $420 plus administrative costs.

Oklahoma (M.D.)

For Information and Application

Carole Smith
Executive Director
State Board of Medical Licensure & Supervision
P.O. Box 18256
Oklahoma City, OK 73154-0256
(405) 848-6841

TO TAKE FLEX (USMG)

All candidates must satisfy the following requirements:

1) Have a medical school diploma and transcript of grades.
2) Have verified all information submitted on application.
3) Make a personal appearance when filing application.

TO TAKE FLEX (FMG)

Same requirements as for USMG with addition of having an ECFMG certificate and certified translation of medical diploma and transcript. Fifth Pathway candidates may apply and will be considered individually in Board meeting. All requirements are subject to approval of the Oklahoma Board.

Acceptable Licensing Exams

1) FLEX.
2) NBME.
3) Other state Board examinations subject to Board discretion.

To Receive State License

Applicants for full licensure must:

(a) Be graduated from a legally chartered medical school, the requirements for graduation from which shall in no way be less than the requirements for graduation from a medical school recognized by the American Medical Association Liaison Council on Medical Education.

(b) Be of good moral character.

(c) Obtain one year of postgraduate training in a facility approved by the Board. The Board does not preapprove the training.

(d) Satisfy other requirements set by the Board.

The Board considers each application individually and meeting the above criteria does not guarantee issuance of a license.

Deadline for FLEX Application
March 27 for the June exam; September 24 for the December exam.

Registration and Exam Fee
FLEX Exam: $400 plus cost of exam.

Oklahoma (D.O.)

For Information and Application

Mary Plender
Oklahoma State Board of Osteopathic Examiners
4848 No. Lincoln Blvd.
Suite 100
Oklahoma City, OK 73105-3321
(405) 528-8625

To Take Exam
All candidates must satisfy the following requirements:

1) Be a graduate of an AOA-approved school of osteopathic medicine.
2) Have completed one year of postgraduate training or the equivalent thereof, in a hospital approved by the Board.
3) Have submitted the application, fees, and all other required items.

Acceptable Licensing Exams

1) NBOE.
2) Oklahoma State Board examination.
3) Reciprocity with other Boards having equal requirements is granted at the discretion of the Board.

To Receive License

Candidate must have passed one of the acceptable licensing exams. The Board may license a candidate by endorsement if the requirements of the state issuing the license are no less stringent than Oklahoma's and the candidate was licensed via a written examination.

Deadline for Exam Application

Two months prior to the exam.

Registration (Annual) and Exam Fees

State Exam: $400.
Licensure Application: $400. (In-State Renewal Fee of $200 each year: $130 Out-of-State Renewal Fee each year by July 1 plus 16 hours of Category 1A-CME each year.)
Dispensing Physician Registration Fee (annual by July 1): $25. (One hour of the 16 hours CME must be on the use of controlled dangerous substances.)

Pass/Fail Rates

1992 results not available.
Note: Oklahoma does not issue a temporary license.

Oregon

For Information and Application

Licensing Department
Physician Program Coordinator
Board of Medical Examiners
620 Crown Plaza
1500 S.W. 1st Ave.
Portland, OR 97201-5826
(503) 229-5770 8:00 a.m.–11:30 a.m. only.

TO TAKE FLEX (USMG)

All candidates must satisfy the following requirements:

1) Must have M.D. or D.O. diploma.
2) Must have completed one year of internship/residency.
3) Must submit application, fees, and other required items.

TO TAKE FLEX (FMG)

Same requirements as for USMG, except candidate must have completed three years of approved progressive internship/residency in the United States in not more than two hospitals and in not more than two specialties. ECFMG/FMGEMS certification is required.

Acceptable Licensing Exams

1) FLEX.
2) NBME.
3) LMCC for U.S. and Canadian graduates only.
4) Written state Board examination that meets Oregon's standards.

To Receive State License

Candidates must have passed one of the acceptable licensing exams and completed required training. License will be issued once application has been completed and candidate has appeared before the Board for a personal interview. If no training or American Board certification or recertification has taken place within the past ten years, candidate is required to take the SPEX, which is a one-day written examination to test the applicant's competency.

Deadline for FLEX Application

75 days prior to the exam.

Registration and Exam Fees

Processing: $270.
Administering: $100.
Components 1 and 2: $420.

SPEX Fees

Processing Fees: $270.
Administering Fee: $100.
SPEX: $240.

Pass/Fail Rates

5 took and passed the June 1992 FLEX exam.

Pennsylvania (M.D.)

For Information and Application

Rita T. Krause
State Board of Medicine
P.O. Box 2649
Harrisburg, PA 17105-2649
(717) 783-1400

TO TAKE FLEX

All candidates must satisfy the following requirements:

1) Completion of an application.
2) Notarized copy of transcript.

Acceptable Licensing Exams

1) FLEX.
2) NBME.
3) Any other state or territorial exam acceptable to the Board.
4) LMCC (passed in or after May 1970).

To Receive State License

1) Candidates must have passed one of the acceptable licensing exams.
2) If training began on or before June 30, 1987, one year of ACGME-approved training is required. If training began on or after July 1, 1987, two years are required for U.S. graduates and three years are required for foreign medical graduates.
3) ECFMG certification is required for foreign medical graduates.
4) Educational requirements must be satisfied by foreign medical graduates.

Note: The FLEX is administered by LGR Examinations, 1315 S. Allen Street, State College, PA 16801, 1-800-877-3926.

Deadline for FLEX Application

90 days prior to the exam.

Registration and Exam Fees

FLEX 1: $280.
FLEX 2: $335.
Both: $490
Application for Licensure (U.S. or Canadian graduates): $20.
Application for Licensure (foreign medical graduates): $80.
Registration Renewal (1991–1992): $80.

Pass/Fail Rates (December 1992 FLEX)

Component 1 only: 244 took the exam; 67.6% passed.
Component 2 only: 465 took the exam; 72.9% passed.
3,475 took Components 1 and 2; 69.8% passed.

Pennsylvania (D.O.)

For Information and Application

John L. Paruso
Administrative Assistant
State Board of Osteopathic Medicine
P.O. Box 2649
Harrisburg, PA 17105-2649
(717) 783-4858

To Take Exam

Pennsylvania does not offer the FLEX for osteopaths. Candidates must take the Pennsylvania State Board exam or the National Boards Parts I, II, and III after they graduate from a school of osteopathic medicine.

Note: For information and application, contact LGR examinations, 1315 South Allen Street, State College, PA 16801; (814) 238-3066.

Acceptable Licensing Exams

1) FLEX.
2) NBOE.
3) Other state Board examinations (if licensed in that state).
4) Pennsylvania State Board exam (75% average required).

To Receive State License

Candidates must have completed one year of an approved osteopathic rotating internship. In addition, they must have passed one of the acceptable written licensing exams and must pass a practical examination in osteopathic manipulative therapy. All candidates applying for a license via endorsement must pass a practical osteopathic manipulative therapy examination.

Deadline for Exam Application

Pennsylvania State Board exam is offered three times a year, in March, June, and November. The Osteopathic Manipulative Therapy exam is offered four times each year, in March, June, September, and November; deadline for both exams is 60 days prior to exam.

Registration and Exam Fees

Osteopathic Manipulative Therapy: $95.
Pennsylvania State Exam: $335.
Pennsylvania Written & OMT Exam: $345.

Puerto Rico

For Information and Application

Board of Medical Examiners
P.O. Box 13969
San Juan, PR 00908
(809) 782-8989
FAX: (809) 782-8733

TO TAKE FLEX (USMG)

All candidates must satisfy the following requirements:

1) Have graduated from a school of medicine accredited by the Puerto Rico Council on Higher Education or the Liaison Committee on Medical Education if the school is located in the United States.
2) Submit an original birth certificate.
3) Submit original certificate of police record or good conduct certificate from the Puerto Rico Police or issued by a competent authority where applicant has resided during the preceding five years.
4) Submit transcript from the institution where the applicant approved premedical courses, obtained a Bachelor of Science degree (B.S.) or courses equivalent to the premedicine curriculum, with a minimum grade point average of 2.5.
5) Submit transcript(s) from institution(s) where applicant completed medical studies.
6) The Dean, Registrar, or other authorized person must certify, at the bottom of the transcript, that the applicant complied totally with the official curriculum courses required to obtain an M.D. degree (basic and clinical sciences).

TO TAKE FLEX (FMG)

1) Same requirements for USMG except that candidate must have graduated from a school recognized by the Puerto Rico Board of Medical Examiners.
2) Applicant must present proof certifying his/her having passed the ECFMG and/or FMGEMS. This evidence must be received by the offices of the Board of Medical Examiners directly from the institution sending it.
3) The Board may demand that any candidate present a certificate of penal record or of good conduct issued by the

competent authority of the country or countries in which the candidate has resided in the subsequent five years.

4) Certification by the Office of Immigration and Naturalization of the U.S. Justice Department indicating that:
   a) Applicant has been granted resident status in the United States or must show that he/she has filed and is processing his/her status as a permanent resident.
   b) Candidate has been a bona fide resident of Puerto Rico during the six months prior to the filing of application.

To Receive Medical License

The Board accepts applications for licensure via FLEX, the NBME, and examination of the Puerto Rico Board of Medical Examiners (given in English or Spanish). To secure a license, candidate must submit same information as when applying for FLEX, including:

1) Two letters attesting to candidate's good moral character by doctors licensed to practice in Puerto Rico.
2) Certification of completion of one year of internship and one year of public service.
3) Submit to an oral examination by the Board.

Deadline and Dates for Exam

The examination of the Board of Puerto Rico is given twice a year, usually in April and November. The deadline for exam applications for the April exam is usually in February and the deadline for the November exam is usually in August.

Registration and Exam Fees

FLEX Component 1: $350.
FLEX Component 2: $400.
Both: $700.

Rhode Island

For Information and Application

Milton W. Hamolsky, M.D.
Chief Administrative Officer
Board of Medical Licensure and Discipline
Rhode Island Department of Health
Cannon Bldg, Rm. 205
Three Capitol Hill

Providence, RI 02908
(401) 277-3855

TO TAKE FLEX (USMG)
All candidates must satisfy the following requirements:

1) Have graduated from an accredited medical school.
2) Have completed one year of internship or residency.

TO TAKE FLEX (FMG)
Same requirements as for USMG with addition of having an ECFMG certificate and completing three years of internship or residency in a U.S. hospital program.

Acceptable Licensing Exams

1) FLEX.
2) NBME.

To Receive State License
Candidates must have passed one of the acceptable licensing exams and appeared for an oral interview before the Board.

Deadline for FLEX Application
100 days prior to the exam.

Registration and Exam Fees
Registration: $350 (if no further examination is required).
Part 1: $220.
Part 2: $275.
Parts 1 and 2: $420 (includes examination fee plus registration fee).

South Carolina

For Information and Application
Annette Brannon
Board of Medical Examiners
1220 Pickins Street
P.O. Box 12245
Columbia, SC 29211
(803) 734-8901

TO TAKE FLEX (USMG)
All candidates must satisfy the following requirements:

1) Be a graduate of an AMA-approved or AOA-approved medical school.

2) Be accepted into a training program in South Carolina, or meet all other licensing criteria, but for FLEX requirement.

TO TAKE FLEX (FMG)

All candidates must satisfy the following requirements:

1) Be a graduate of an approved medical school.
2) Have an ECFMG permanent certificate.
3) Be accepted into training program in South Carolina, or meet all other licensing criteria, but for FLEX requirement.

Acceptable Licensing Exams

1) FLEX.
2) NBME.
3) NBOE.
4) SPEX.

To Receive State License

Candidates must have passed one of the acceptable licensing exams. SPEX is required if FLEX or National Board has not been passed in the past ten years, or if not Board-certified or recertified within the past ten years. A personal appearance before the entire Board is required for FMGs, and a personal appearance before an individual Board member or before full Board is required for USMGs.

Deadline for FLEX Application

90 days prior to the exam.

Registration and Exam Fees

FLEX: $600.
Reregistration: $80 annually.

South Dakota

For Information and Application

Robert D. Johnson
Executive Secretary
Bd. of Medical & Osteopathic Examiners
1323 S. Minnesota Ave.
Sioux Falls, SD 57105
(605) 336-1965

TO TAKE FLEX (USMG)
All candidates must satisfy the following requirements:

1) Have a medical school or osteopathic school diploma.
2) Have completed or be enrolled in an approved residency in the United States or Canada.
3) Must present candidate's original credentials before a Board member.

TO TAKE FLEX (FMG)
Same requirements as for USMG with addition of having an ECFMG certificate and being, or having completed the form Declaration of Intention to become, a U.S. citizen.

Acceptable Licensing Exams

1) FLEX.
2) NMBE.
3) May accept Canadian examinations and individual state Board examinations on an individual basis.

To Receive State License
For licensure by examination, each candidate must appear prior to the exam and present his original credentials to a Board member and at the Board office. He must subsequently pass FLEX. For licensure by reciprocity or endorsement via the NBME, each candidate must appear at the office of the Board and before one member of the Board.

Deadline for FLEX Application
April 1 for the June exam; September 15 for the December exam.

Registration and Exam Fees
Each Component: $275.
Both: $550.

Pass/Fail Rates
3 took and failed the December 1992 FLEX exam.

Tennessee (M.D.)
For Information and Application
Sylvia Wright
Administrator
Board of Medical Examiners
283 Plus Park Blvd.

Nashville, TN 37247-1010
(615) 367-6393

TO TAKE FLEX (USMG)
All candidates must satisfy the following requirements:

1) Be a graduate of an LCGME-approved medical school in the United States or Canada.
2) Submit three notarized recent photographs.
3) Be of good moral character.

TO TAKE FLEX (FMG)
All candidates must satisfy the following requirements:

1) Submit copy of medical school transcript (in English).
2) Submit evidence of legal residence in the United States if not a U.S. citizen.
3) Have ECFMG certification.
4) Be of good moral character.
5) Prior to licensure, must complete a three-year continuous residency program.

Acceptable Licensing Exams

1) FLEX.
2) NBME.
3) LMCC.
4) Written state Board exams prior to 1972.

To Receive State License
Must have passed one of the acceptable licensing exams and completed one year of a residency program. All FMGs are required to have an interview with at least one Board member and to demonstrate minimal competence in conversational English. FMGs also must complete a three-year continuous residency program. Fifth Pathway program candidates must document their enrollment in a medical training program prior to July 1, 1982, U.S. citizenship at the time of enrollment, and the completion of all training requirements except internship and social service. Reciprocity is considered on an individual basis.

Deadline for FLEX Application
90 days prior to the exam.

Registration and Exam Fees
Component 1: $270.
Component 2: $325.

Both: $470.
All fees include a nonrefundable application fee of $50.)

Tennessee (D.O.)

For Information and Application

Anita Vantries
Administrative Manager
Board of Osteopathic Examination
283 Plus Park Blvd.
Nashville, TN 37247-1010
(615) 367-6393

TO TAKE EXAM

All candidates must be graduates of a school of osteopathic medicine, and complete an internship.

The Board offers a specific exam for D.O. candidates.

To Receive State License

Candidates must pass a specific exam given by the National Board.

Fees

Application (nonrefundable): $95.
Examination: $200.
Reciprocity: $200.
Renewal: $250 (Biennially).
State Regulatory Fee: $5 (Annually).
Exemption for Intern, Resident, or Fellow: $10.
Late Renewal Penalty: $100.
Duplicate License: $25.
Limited X-Ray Technical Application (nonrefundable): $75.

Texas

For Information and Application

Homer R. Goehrs, M.D.
Executive Director
Board of Medical Examiners
P.O. Box 149134
Austin, TX 78714-9134
(512) 834-7728

TO TAKE FLEX (USMG)

All candidates must satisfy the following requirements:

1) Be a graduate of an LCME- or AOA-approved medical school.
2) Be 21 years of age and of good professional character.
3) Have completed 60 semester hours of college courses other than in medical school.

TO TAKE FLEX (FMG)

Same requirements as for USMG with addition of having an ECFMG certificate. In addition, three years of training in one field of medicine in a program approved by the Board are required for candidates who are not graduates of approved schools. A candidate must be eligible for licensure to practice medicine in the country in which the candidate's school of graduation is located.

Acceptable Licensing Exams

1) FLEX.
2) NBME.
3) NBOE.
4) LMCC.
5) Other state Board exams.

Note: Items 2 to 5 apply to reciprocity applicants only. Applicant must pass SPEX unless American specialty Board-certified or recertified within the past ten years.

To Receive State License

Candidates must have passed one of the acceptable licensing exams and must have passed the Texas Medical Jurisprudence Examination. USMGs must have completed one year of graduate medical training approved by the Board: FMGs must have completed three years approved by the Board. A personal interview is required. The Board grants licenses via reciprocal endorsement and examination.

Deadline for FLEX Application

February 1 for the June exam; July 30 for the December exam.

Registration and Exam Fees

FLEX: $800.

Annual registration fee: $292.

Pass/Fail Rates (June 1992 FLEX)

Component 1: 95% passed.
Component 2: 97% passed.

Utah (M.D.)

For Information and Application

Diane Blake
Bureau Manager
Health Care Professions
Div. of Occupational & Professional Licensing
160 E. 300 South
P.O. Box 45805
Salt Lake City, UT 84145-0805
(801) 530-6628

To Take FLEX (USMG)

All candidates must satisfy the following requirements:

1) FLEX application.
2) Have a LCME-accredited medical school diploma.
3) ECFMG if foreign medical graduate or FMGEMS if Fifth Pathway.

Acceptable Licensing Exams

1) FLEX.
2) NBME.
3) Other written state Board exams.
4) USMLE

To Receive State License

Candidates must have passed one or an approved combination of acceptable licensing exams, plus have completed an LCME-accredited postgraduate education program of at least one year. The Board has the right to require any physician applying for licensure by endorsement who has been in practice for more than 10 years to pass Component 2 of FLEX or the SPEX before licensure is granted. A personal appearance before the Board may be required.

Deadline for FLEX Application

March 1 for the June exam; September 1 for the December exam.

Registration and Exam Fees

Filing Fee: $60.
Component 1: $240.
Component 2: $325.
Both: $470.

Utah (D.O.)

For Information and Application

Bureau Manager
Health Care Professions
Div. of Occ. & Prof. Licensing
160 E. 300 South
P.O. Box 45805
Salt Lake City, UT 84145-0805
(801) 530-6628

TO TAKE FLEX (USMG)

All candidates must satisfy the following requirements:

1) FLEX application.
2) Have a medical school diploma.

TO TAKE FLEX (FMG)

Same requirements as for USMG with the addition of the following:

1) A current ECFMG certificate.
2) If candidate has been out of postgraduate training for more than two years, he must submit evidence of CME activity.

Acceptable Licensing Exams

1) FLEX.
2) NBME.
3) Other written state Board exams.
4) USMLE

To Receive State License

Candidates must have passed one of the acceptable licensing exams, plus have completed an LCME-accredited postgraduate education program of at least one year. The Board has the right to require any physician applying for licensure by endorsement who has been in practice for more than 10 years to pass Component 2 of FLEX or SPEX before licensure is granted. A personal appearance before the Board may be required. Any osteopathic physician licensed by FLEX must come before the Board for an oral interview.

Deadline for FLEX Application

March 1 for the June exam; September 1 for the December exam.

Registration and Exam Fees

Filing Fee: $150 (which is applied toward a Utah state license).
Controlled Substance: $90.
FLEX: $470.

Vermont (M.D.)

For Information and Application

Debbie Morehouse
Staff Assistant
Board of Medical Practice
Secretary of State's Office
109 State Street
Montpelier, VT 05609-1106
(802) 828-2673

TO TAKE FLEX (USMG)

All candidates must satisfy the following requirements:

1) Must have graduated from a school of medicine.
2) Have completed one year of ACGME-approved postgraduate training (internship or residency).

TO TAKE FLEX (FMG)

Same requirements as for USMG with addition of having an ECFMG certificate. Fifth Pathway programs are not acceptable for postgraduate training requirement.

Acceptable Licensing Exams

1) FLEX.
2) NBME.

To Receive State License (USMG)

Candidates must have passed one of the acceptable licensing exams, completed the application process, one year of postgraduate training in an ACGME-approved program, and made a personal appearance before a Board member.

To Receive State License (FMG)

Candidate must have passed one of the acceptable licensing exams and FMGEMS, complete application process, three years of postgraduate education in ACGME-approved program, and a personal appearance before a Board member. Contact Board for more information.

Deadline for FLEX Application
March 25 for the June exam; September 20 for the December exam.

Registration and Exam Fees
Component 1: $360.
Component 2: $415.
Both: $560.
License Application: $190.
Verification Fee: $20.

Vermont (D.O.)
For Information and Application
Nancy Basaldu
Board of Osteopathic Physicians and Surgeons
Secretary of State's Office
109 State Street
Montpelier, VT 05609-1106
(802) 828-2191

Acceptable Licensing Exams
1) FLEX only with extra section on osteopathic practice and principles. Contact Board office regarding State exam.
2) NBOE.

To Receive State License
Candidates must have passed one of the acceptable licensing exams. Reciprocity is granted if candidate is a graduate of an accredited school of osteopathy and has practiced in another state for five years under a valid license. The standards of the state in which the license was granted must be equal to those of Vermont.

Application and Exam Fees
Application: $50.
Initial License: $20.
FLEX: $545.

Virginia
For Information and Application
Eugenia K. Dorson
Deputy Executive Director

State Board of Medicine
6606 West Board Street, 4th Floor
Richmond, VA 23230-1717
(804) 662-9908

TO TAKE FLEX (USMG)
All candidates must satisfy the following requirements:

1) Have a valid medical school diploma.
2) Have one year of internship/residency in a U.S. or Canadian AMA-approved program.

TO TAKE FLEX (FMG)
Must have three years of internship/residency in a U.S. or Canadian AMA-approved program with addition of having an ECFMG certificate. Fifth Pathway candidates may be accepted if they meet FMG requirements.

Acceptable Licensing Exams

1) FLEX or AOA.
2) NBME.
3) LMCC.
4) Other written state Board exams taken before 1970.
5) Other written state Board exams taken any year in addition to being American Board certified.

To Receive State License
Candidates must have passed one of the acceptable licensing exams. The Board will not accept FLEX candidates who have failed the exam three times via endorsement. Candidates may sit for three additional times upon completion of one additional year of approved training.

Deadline for FLEX Application
75 days prior to the date of exam.

Registration and Exam Fees
Component 1: $275.
Component 2: $325.
Both: $600.
Upon successful passing of the FLEX, the applicant shall pay a fee of $125 for licensure.

Virgin Islands
For Information and Application
Secundina Mercado, M.D.
Secretary

Board of Medical Examiners
Department of Health
48 Sugar Estate
Charlotte Amalie
St. Thomas, VI 00802
(809) 774-0117 or 776-8311, ext. 201 or 203

TO TAKE FLEX (USMG)

All candidates must satisfy the following requirements:

1) At time of application, candidate must also submit a chronological account of time spent between graduation and application.
2) Submit an autographed (on back), passport-size photograph of self.
3) Be a graduate of an accredited school of medicine and submit attesting document.
4) Have completed one year of internship in a hospital recognized by the AMA and submit attesting documents.
5) Be at least 21 years old (birth certificate or similar evidence necessary).
6) Be of good moral character (two currently dated letters of character reference, one preferably from Director of training program, attesting to above).
7) Must not be addicted to intemperate use of alcohol, stimulants, or narcotic drugs. Affidavit attesting to the above, signed by applicant, is necessary.

TO TAKE FLEX (FMG)

Same requirements as for USMG with addition of having a valid ECFMG certificate or a Fifth Pathway program certificate.

Acceptable Licensing Exams

1) FLEX.

FLEX is administered as the state licensing exam. On passing, applicants are required to submit themselves to an oral interview.

To Receive State License

Candidates must have passed written and oral components.

Deadline for FLEX Application

12 weeks prior to exam date.

Registration and Exam Fees

Both Components: $500.

Annual License Registration: $200.

Washington (M.D.)

For Information and Application

Beverly A. Gifford
Program Manager
Board of Medical Examiners
Dept. of Health
1300 Quince Street
P.O. Box 47866
Olympia, WA 98504-7866
(206) 753-2205

To Take Exam

All candidates must satisfy the following requirements:

1) Graduate from a medical school approved by the Board.
2) Have completed at least nine months of postgraduate training in an AMA-accredited program or Canadian-approved postgraduate training program.
3) Obtain four hours of AIDS education.
4) Obtain standard certificate of ECFMG.

Acceptable Licensing Exams

1) NBME.
2) FLEX Components 1 and 2 with passing score of 75.
3) Endorsement of state exams, except from Florida and Hawaii.

To Receive State License

Candidates must pass FLEX or the NBME or have endorsement of state exam, except from Florida and Hawaii; have an indefinite ECFMG certificate; complete one year of postgraduate training if graduated from medical school before July 1, 1985, or two years of postgraduate training if after July 1, 1985.

Deadline for FLEX Application

March 1 for the June exam: September 1 for the December exam.

Registration and Exam Fees

Endorsement Application: $325.

FLEX Component 1 and 2 exam: $625.

FLEX Component 1: $325.
FLEX Component 2: $345.

Pass/Fail Rates (June 1992 FLEX)
22 took the exam; 17 passed.

Washington (D.O.)

For Information and Application

Shannon Walker
Representative
Board of Osteopathic Medicine and Surgery
Professional Licensing Services
1300 Quince St.
P.O. Box 47870
Olympia, WA 98504-7870
(206) 586-5962

To Take Exam
All candidates must satisfy the following requirements:

1) Graduate of AOA-approved school of osteopathic medicine.
2) Have completed one year of postgraduate training in an AOA- or AMA-accredited hospital program.
3) Obtain seven hours of AIDS education.

Acceptable Licensing Exams

1) NBOE.
2) FLEX and Washington exam in osteopathic practices and principles.
3) Endorsement of state exams that include a section on osteopathic practices and principles.

To Receive License
Candidates must pass FLEX and the Washington written exam in osteopathic practices and principles or must pass the NBOE or have endorsement of state exam that included a section on osteopathic practices and principles.

Deadline for Exam Application
For the FLEX: February 1 for the June exam: August 1 for the December exam. For the Washington written exam: scheduled individually.

Registration and Exam Fees

Endorsement Application: $500.
FLEX/State Exam: $600.
Endorsement FLEX/State Exam: $500

West Virginia (M.D.)

For Information and Application

For FLEX: Lona Skiles
For Licensure: Nancy Clay
Board of Medicine
101 Dee Drive
Charleston, WV 25311
(304) 558-2921

TO TAKE FLEX (USMG)

All candidates must have graduated from a medical school approved by the Board.

TO TAKE FLEX (FMG)

Same requirements as for USMG with addition of having an ECFMG certificate or scores with letter stating its validity. The Board recognizes Fifth Pathway programs.

Acceptable Licensing Exams

1) FLEX.
2) NBME.
3) Written state Board exams.
4) LMCC.

To Receive State License

Candidates must have passed one of the acceptable licensing exams, be interviewed by a Board member, and meet all other requirements. If an American, Canadian, or Puerto Rican graduate, must have completion of at least one year of postgraduate clinical training in the United States or Canada, or if foreign medical graduate other than outlined above, must have completion of at least three years of postgraduate clinical training in the United States or Canada and have a valid ECFMG.

Deadline for FLEX Application

March 1 for the June exam; September 1 for the December exam.

Registration and Exam Fees

Component 1: $300.
Component 2: $350.
Both: $600.

Pass/Fail Rates (June 1992 Exam)

33 took Components 1 and 2; 11 passed both; none passed Component 1 only; 4 passed Component 2 only. 31 took Component 1 only; 10 passed. 10 took Component 2 only; 7 passed.

West Virginia (D.O.)

For Information and Application

Cheryl D. Schreiber
Assistant Secretary
Board of Osteopathy
334 Penco Road
Weirton, WV 26062
(304) 723-4638

To Take Exam

All candidates must satisfy the following requirements:

1) Have a diploma from a professional school or college of osteopathy recognized by the AOA or the Board.
2) Have completed one year of AOA-approved internship.
3) Must be at least 18 years old and be of good moral character.

Acceptable Licensing Exams

1) West Virginia State Board exam.
2) NBOE.

To Receive State License

All candidates must pass one of the acceptable licensing exams and complete all other licensing requirements. Candidates for endorsement via NBOE must submit transcript of grades and NBOE certificate. The Board has reciprocal agreements with many states and may issue a license without examination. The candidate must have met the legal requirements equal to requirements in force in West Virginia at the time license was received. For reciprocity or endorsement, the candidate must meet with the Board before license is issued.

Deadline for Exam

Regular examinations are held twice yearly at the Board's discretion. The dates are published in *The Journal of the American*

Osteopathic Association; applications are due 90 days prior to the exam date. The exam is a two-day written text covering anatomy, physiology, biochemistry, pharmacology, pathology, microbiology and public health, surgery, ob/gyn, pediatrics, neurology, psychiatry, and osteopathic principles.

Registration and Exam Fee
Exam: $325.

Wisconsin

For Information and Application

Patricia Schenck (Application)
Program Assistant
Deanna Zychowski (Information)
Administrative Assistant
Dept. of Regulation & Licensing
Medical Examining Board
P.O. Box 8935
Madison, WI 53708
(608) 266-2811

TO TAKE FLEX (USMG)

All candidates must satisfy the following requirements:

1) Have a medical school diploma.
2) Have completed one year of postgraduate training in an approved facility in the United States or Canada.

TO TAKE FLEX (FMG)

Same requirements as for USMG with addition of having an ECFMG certificate or scores with letter stating its validity. The Board recognizes Fifty Pathway programs.

Acceptable Licensing Exams

1) FLEX.
2) NBME/NBOE.
3) Endorsement of state Board exam taken before 1972.
4) LMCC taken after January 1, 1978.

To Receive State License

Candidates must have passed one of the acceptable licensing exams and may have to appear before the Board for an oral examination. The Board maintains no reciprocity with other states.

Deadline for FLEX Application
Three months prior to the exam.

Registration and Exam Fees
Both Components: $460.

Pass/Fail Rates (June 1992 FLEX)
37 took Component 1; 34 passed. 38 took Component 2; 35 passed.

Wyoming

For Information and Application

Carole Shotwell
Executive Secretary
Board of Medicine
Barrett Bldg., Second Floor
Cheyenne, WY 82002
(307) 777-6463

TO TAKE FLEX (USMG)
All candidates must satisfy the following requirements:

1) Have a medical diploma from an accredited medical or osteopathic school.
2) Submit three letters of recommendation.

TO TAKE FLEX (FMG)
Same requirements as for USMG with addition of having an ECFMG certificate, two years of on-campus medical education, and two years of postgraduate training in an ACGME- or AOA-accredited program.

Acceptable Licensing Exams

1) FLEX.
2) NBME.
3) NBOE.
4) LMCC.
5) USMLE

To Receive State License
Candidates must have passed one of the acceptable licensing exams, appeared for an oral interview before the Board (offered February, June, and October), and have one year of postgraduate training in an ACGME- or AOA-accredited program for U.S. graduates and two years for FMGs.

Deadline for FLEX Application
90 days prior to the exam.

Registration and Exam Fees

Component 1: $280.
Component 2: $335.
Both: $615.
License Fee: $250.

Pass/Fail Rates (June 1992 Exam)
1 candidate took the December 1992 exam and passed.

Note: This guide is intended to help you take the first steps toward becoming licensed, and it is the responsibility of the reader to contact the individual state Boards for complete requirements.

ECFMG Examination Fees

Fees for the July 13–14, 1993, Foreign Medical Graduate Examination in the Medical Sciences (FMGEMS) are:

- Basic Medical Science Component (Day 1 only)—$275.
- Clinical Science Component and ECFMG English Test (Day 2 only)—$275.
- Basic Medical Science Component, Clinical Science Component, and ECFMG English Test (Days 1 and 2)—$450.

The fee for the ECFMG English Test and the fee for the Test of English as a Foreign Language (TOEFL) acceptance have increased to $30. Other examination-related services remain the same.

Appendix 5.2

Endorsement and Reciprocity Policies of State Boards

True reciprocity, or the automatic mutual exchange of licensing privileges, has generally become obsolete. Although certain states may have the same requirements for licensure, reciprocity usually is not automatic or guaranteed. Instead, most states now issue licenses by endorsement. Endorsement is the issuing of a license to practice medicine to a candidate from another state following the submission of the applicant's original FLEX or National Board scores and the filing of an endorsement application by the candidate in the state he or she chooses. The applicant also must meet those requirements not necessarily mandatory in his or her own state. For example, certain states may require an interview with the licensing Board or an oral exam, whereas other states may require more than one year of graduate medical education. The public has sought immunity against an increasing number of unethical physicians over the past several years. Therefore, many states have changed or amended their policies regarding reciprocity and have instated more stringent requirements and restrictions. Implementation of these restrictions also tends to discourage a concentration of physicians in prime or highly desirable areas.

Alabama—Maintains reciprocity with all states, providing applicant meets all requirements, but will not accept Florida State Board (will reciprocate with Florida if candidate took FLEX).

Alaska—No reciprocity. License may be obtained through endorsement, and candidate also must meet all state requirements.

Arizona (M.D.)—No reciprocity. License may be obtained through endorsement of last exam, i.e., FLEX or National Board. Candidates also must meet state requirements. If candidate's last written exam was taken more than 10 years preceding the application, the SPEX exam also must be taken.

Arizona (D.O.)—Maintains reciprocity with all states.

Arkansas—Maintains reciprocity with all states except Florida.

California (M.D.)—To be licensed, applicants who meet the minimum education requirements, have passed an approved licensing exam, and have completed at least one year of ACGME-approved postgraduate training may be eligible for licensure. Applicants who have been certified by the National Board for five years or more, or other applicants who have practiced medicine in another state for four years or more, must meet the minimum education requirements and may be required to pass a reciprocity written exam (SPEX), an oral exam, or both.

California (D.O.)—Reciprocity is granted if the candidate holds an unrestricted license in osteopathic medicine in another state whose written licensing exam is recognized and approved by the Board. Candidates must still pass the oral/practical exam of the California Board.

Colorado—No reciprocity. Candidates must meet all state requirements.

Connecticut—No reciprocity. Candidates must meet all state requirements.

Delaware—No reciprocity. Candidates must meet all state requirements.

District of Columbia—License by endorsement only.

Florida (M.D.)—Florida does not offer licensure via reciprocity, only via examination or endorsement.

Florida (D.O.)—Licensure by endorsement. All applicants must meet current state requirements. Applicants must have taken all three parts of the NBOME or another state Board exam that is similar to or more difficult than the Florida State Board exam and that has an osteopathic component. The Board does not accept FLEX.

Georgia—Georgia does not offer true reciprocity. All applicants must meet state requirements. The Board endorses the FLEX,

National Boards, National Osteopathic Boards, and older State Board examinations except for the following states: Arizona, California, Connecticut, District of Columbia, Florida, Hawaii, Illinois, New Hampshire, New York, Puerto Rico, Utah, and Wisconsin.

Guam—No reciprocity. Candidates must meet all state requirements.

Hawaii (M.D.)—No reciprocity. Candidates must meet all state requirements.

Hawaii (D.O.)—Reciprocity granted with states having similar requirements. License by endorsement and by meeting all state requirements.

Idaho—No reciprocity. Will endorse USMLE, FLEX, state Board exam, or National Board exam as long as license is current.

Illinois—No reciprocity. License is granted on an individual basis by endorsement. Candidates also must meet all state licensure requirements.

Indiana—Maintains reciprocity with all states.

Iowa—License by endorsement only. No straight reciprocity licensure granted.

Kansas—License by endorsement only.

Kentucky—License by endorsement only.

Louisiana—Reciprocity with all states except Alaska, Florida, Hawaii, Puerto Rico, and Canada, except on the basis of successful passage of FLEX or the National Boards. All three parts must be passed to receive a reciprocal license. D.O. licensure by successful passage of FLEX. Additional requirements for FMGs.

Maine (M.D.)—No reciprocity. Will endorse USMLE, National Boards, FLEX, or state exam certified as passed in another jurisdiction.

Maine (D.O.)—No reciprocity. Will endorse National Boards, FLEX, or state exam. FLEX applicants will need to pass an exam in osteopathic practices and principles.

Maryland—No reciprocity. Candidates must meet all state requirements.

Massachusetts—No reciprocity. Candidates must meet all state requirements.

Michigan (M.D.)—License by endorsement only. Applicant must have a current, active license in another state.

Michigan (D.O.)—License by endorsement only.

Minnesota—License by endorsement only. Candidate also must meet state requirements. If ten years have passed since initial licensing exam, candidate must pass SPEX, unless currently specialty Board-certified. Foreign medical graduates must pass ECFMG exam.

Mississippi—Licence by endorsement only.

Missouri—Does not have direct reciprocity with any state. Candidates must meet all state requirements.

Montana—Maintains reciprocity with all states, except Florida.

Nebraska—Licensure is granted on an individualized basis by endorsement only. Applicant also must meet all state requirements.

Nevada (M.D.)—License by endorsement only. Candidates also must have three years of residency and meet all other requirements for licensure.

Nevada (D.O.)—Will endorse National Boards or written state exam. A personal oral interview is required. A one-year, AOA-approved internship or a three-year, AMA or AOA residency program is required.

New Hampshire—License by endorsement only.

New Jersey—No reciprocity. The Board will accept a FLEX examination taken prior to June 1985 if the individual received a FLEX weighted average of 75 or higher using scores from the last examination taken. A score of 75 or higher is required in each component of the new FLEX taken after December 1984. The Board accepts a National Board examination as the basis for licensure regardless of the date taken. Individual state licensing examinations are accepted only if taken prior to January 1, 1973.

New Mexico (M.D.)—License by endorsement or examination only.

New Mexico (D.O.)—No reciprocity. Will endorse FLEX, original state Board exam with requirements equal to New Mexico, or National Board exam. The Board meets quarterly, and an oral interview with the Board is required.

New York—License by endorsement only.

North Carolina—License by endorsement only.

North Dakota—Reciprocity is granted to a state medical license holder whose license was obtained via a written state Board examination or FLEX taken in that state. Holders of NBME or LMCC certification are granted a license based on endorsement. Each physician also must meet the licensure requirements regarding residency training. An oral interview before the Board is required.

Ohio—Will endorse National Board or LMCC (will not endorse or transfer FLEX), or must have current unrestricted license in another state.

Oklahoma (M.D.)—Application for license may be based on endorsement of a state license, licensure obtained in Canada, Great Britain, or territory of the United States, FLEX exam scores, National Board scores; at the discretion of the Board.

Oklahoma (D.O.)—A license is granted at the Board's discretion (FLEX not accepted).

Oregon—Oregon reciprocates with all states except Alaska, Florida, and Hawaii. However, if the FLEX examination is taken in those states, according to Oregon standards, reciprocity would be considered on an individual basis. For all states where the FLEX examination is taken, reciprocity is considered only if the FLEX examination meets Oregon standards and requirements. All licensing requirements must be met.

Pennsylvania (M.D.)—License by endorsement only.

Pennsylvania (D.O.)—License by endorsement only if other state reciprocates.

Puerto Rico—The Board accepts applications for licensure via FLEX, the NBME, and examination of the Puerto Rico Board of Medical Examiners (given in English or Spanish).

Rhode Island—Endorsement based on FLEX and National Boards or state Boards that reciprocate with Rhode Island.

South Carolina—License by endorsement only.

South Dakota—For licensure by reciprocity or endorsement via the NBME, each candidate must appear at the office of the Board and before one member of the Board.

Tennessee (M.D.)—Reciprocity is not automatic but is considered on an individual basis.

Tennessee (D.O.)—Reciprocates on an individual basis with any other state if candidate means all other state requirements.

Texas—The Board grants licenses via reciprocal endorsement and examination.

Utah (M.D.)—The Board has the right to require any physician applying for licensure by reciprocity who has been in practice for more than 15 years to take Component 2 of FLEX before licensure may be granted.

Utah (D.O.)—No reciprocity. License by endorsement only.

Vermont (M.D.)—License by endorsement only.

Vermont (D.O.)—Reciprocity is granted if the candidate is a graduate of an accredited school of osteopathy and has practiced in another state for five years under a valid license. The standards of the state in which the license was granted must be equal to those of Vermont.

Virginia—License by endorsement only.

Virgin Islands—No reciprocity or endorsement with United States. Candidates must pass FLEX exam administered in Virgin Islands and meet all state requirements.

Washington (M.D.)—No reciprocity. Will endorse FLEX or National Board Exam or state exams except from Florida and Hawaii.

Washington (D.O.)—No reciprocity. License by endorsement only.

West Virginia (M.D.)—Maintains reciprocity with all states provided candidate has passed one of the acceptable licensing exams and meets all other requirements. Candidate also must be interviewed by a Board member.

West Virginia (D.O.)—For reciprocity or endorsement, the candidate must meet with the Board before license is issued. The applicant must meet all licensing requirements.

Wisconsin—No reciprocity. License by endorsement only.

Wyoming—The Board may grant a license by endorsement provided the candidate holds a license from another state, his or her qualifications are in no way less than those required by Wyoming, and the candidate passes an interview with the Board.

Chapter 6

Office Design, Structure, and Equipment

GOALS

The goals of this chapter are to present the basic design considerations for a medical office, and list all the equipment and supplies that might be needed for a medical office.

PART 1

Office Design and Layout Considerations

If you are joining a preestablished medical group that already has an office for you, you may not need to consider many of the items detailed in this chapter. However, you might want to modify the structure or layout of the office space you will be assigned, in which case many of the same considerations would apply as in designing an office from scratch. Consider these general features in designing an office:

1. Type of medical practice
2. Size/patient load of the medical practice
3. Need for support facilities and structures
4. Age/culture of patients served
5. Size/type of support staff
6. Possible need for new or different equipment
7. Need or ability to expand the space and/or services in the future

Minimum Features

1. Entry/waiting area (2 chairs minimum)
2. Registration/business desk
3. Examination room

The absolute minimal square footage for this spartan office arrangement would be about 150 square feet (7 × 21 feet in dimensions). Most independent solo practitioner offices, however, require at least 1200 square feet of floor space. See Appendix 6.1 for some sample design layouts for small-sized offices.

More Features

A more complete list of the standard medical office structure components would include the following features:

1. Entryway
2. Reception/waiting room
3. Greeting/appointment desk
4. Billing/collection desk
5. Examination room(s)
6. Storage area for medical records
7. Physician's office
8. Staff lounge/conference room
9. Nurses' station
10. Restroom(s)
11. Coat closet for staff

Additional or "optional" rooms may be needed (depending on the specialty):

1. Cast/splint room with materials storage area
2. "Subwaiting room" (this is often needed in ophthalmologist's offices to have a low light waiting area for patients who have had their pupils dilated or if patients will be waiting for results of lab tests or x-rays)
3. Surgical suite/operating room/procedure room
4. X-ray room with film developing area or closet
5. Physician dictation area or computer terminal work area
6. Physical or occupational therapy room
7. Laboratory
8. ECG/echocardiography/ultrasound room
9. On-call room with sleeping accommodations if the physician has to take overnight call from the office
10. Pharmaceutical preparation and/or storage room

Parking

Do not forget to make allowance for adequate parking for your patients. In planning the parking area for your office, the first thing to do is to figure out how many parking spaces you will need. In general, there should be one parking space for delivery trucks, one for the physician, one for each staff member who will be present in the office at the same time, and then additional spaces for the patients. To determine the number of patient spaces needed, a simple formula states that the number of parking spaces should equal the number of patients seen per hour times the average number of hours the patient spends in the office. At a minimum, there should be spaces for the number of patients seen in an hour even if the average patient stay is less than hour, so as to accommodate overlapping time slots for patients.

You may need to separately and clearly mark the spaces reserved for yourself and your office staff if the number of parking spaces available for the practice is "tight." At least one space must be designated and clearly marked for handicapped parking, and this should be the space closest to the office door or access ramp. If your office does not have either the space or adjacent land for its own parking lot, you will need to make some kind of arrangements with a nearby lot or garage for parking for your patients.

In planning your parking lot, just as for the office building itself, you need to determine if there are any specific local building codes that apply to parking lot sizes or set back distances. In the overall design of your office, you should consider whether you want to have the parking on ground level adjacent to the building, on ground level with the office portion of the building directly above the parking lot, or have parking spaces below ground underneath the office. Obviously, the cost of ground level parking adjacent to the building is cheaper than for ground level spaces directly beneath the building, which, in turn, is somewhat cheaper than having to excavate for parking spots below ground level beneath the building. In designing the parking lot, you will need to decide if the parking spaces will be set parallel, diagonal, or perpendicular to the curb or border of the lot. Diagonally set parking spaces are the easiest for people to drive into and back out of, but end up wasting "corner" space at either end of the lot. Parallel parking spaces are best to use in a narrow access area but are the most difficult for patients to get into and out of. Perpendicular parking spaces are in some ways the most efficient. If there are two rows of parking spaces, as well as two-way traffic to access these spaces, the total width of the parking space required will be 65 feet. This width can be narrowed only by about 3 feet if only one-way traffic access to the parking lot is allowed.

To plan the design of your parking lot, you may want to cut out some squares of paper scaled appropriately to the size of a single parking space and maneuver these around on a scaled piece of paper representing the parking lot to determine the most efficient use of the space available. In general, for parallel parking against the curb, each car space should be 9 feet × 24 feet. For perpendicular parking, each space should be 9 feet × 20 feet at a minimum, but often a 10-foot width per space is better to allow easier car door opening. For diagonal parking, if each space is set at a 45 degree angle to the curb, a distance of about 14 feet along the curb for each space will be needed and a depth of 20 feet from the curb. If you specifically designate one section of the parking lot for compact cars and clearly mark this, the above footage requirements per space can be reduced somewhat. If, for whatever reason, a number of your patients drive motorcycles, you could make several much smaller spaces for motorcycle parking and thereby not take up full-sized spaces.

Design

There are general guidelines to follow in designing your office building or suite:

1. Make certain that your design is in accordance with local building codes and fire codes (which may have specific limitations regarding different room sizes, access corridor lengths, building materials or style, water sprinklers, and smoke detectors).
2. Make sure your design is in accordance with the Federal requirements of the "Americans with Disabilities Act" passed in 1991. This act requires even small businesses to make "reasonable accommodations" to allow patients with disabilities equal access to facilities (such as medical offices) and services. The specific requirements mandated by this act have not been completely determined at the time of writing of this book. The features that are expected to be required are assurance that all rooms are accessible by wheelchair and that restrooms are large enough to accommodate wheelchair patients. Information on this Federal law's requirements is obtainable from the U.S. Justice Department Civil Rights

Division (202–514–0301). See Appendix A at the end of the book for additional sources of information on the details of this act.

3. The office area and rooms should be planned in such a fashion that future modifications of the layout to allow for expansion of the practice or addition of new equipment will not be difficult.
4. Floors and walls in the patient care areas should be easily cleanable if you see pediatric patients, patients with infectious diseases, or perform any procedures where blood or body fluids may be spilled (thus vinyl sheeting, gloss paints, or other smooth-finish surfaces may be preferable to cloth-type surfaces for ease of cleaning).
5. Ensure adequate protection of patient privacy. This often entails very careful planning of whether doors open into or out of rooms. In addition, extra sound insulation should be provided for all the patient rooms so that your interviews and conversations with patients cannot be heard by people in other rooms.
6. There should be an area for the office staff that allows them some privacy from the patients in the office (for the staff's meal breaks and rest periods). New OSHA (Occupational Safety and Health Administration) regulations, in fact, require that all food and beverage consumption be in a separate area away from the patient care areas (to prevent any potential body fluid contamination of foods or beverages).
7. Allow for extra electrical outlets beyond the number required by building codes. It is much easier to have them placed with the initial construction than to have them added later.

Specific Design Considerations

Reception/waiting room. Generally, waiting room size should be 10 square feet of floor space per patient seen per hour, or enough space for two to three times the number of chairs as the number of patients normally seen in an hour. This extra allowance for chairs is to accommodate family members and other people who would accompany or assist a patient to the office. Most of the waiting area should be directly visible from either the sign-in desk or a nurse's desk to monitor the waiting room for patients who might be developing some form of distress. If you see pediatric patients or if a number of your patients bring their children with them to office visits, having a separate play area in the waiting room is often greatly appreciated by the patients. The best designs for this include a 3- to 4-foot high, clear (Plexiglass or clear plastic) wall around the area so that it is physically separated from the rest of the room, but the parents and/or nurses can observe the children while they are in the play area. Toys selected for the play area should be carefully chosen, avoiding ones with (aspiratable) small parts, ones that make a lot of noise, and ones that are hard to clean.

Somewhere in the waiting room there should be a coat rack and/or coat closet for patients and persons accompanying them. In general, separate chairs are preferred in waiting rooms instead of couches or benches. This is because most patients do not want to sit in close physical proximity to other patients in the office. Mirrors should generally not be placed in waiting rooms, as most patients who feel ill do not want to have to look at themselves in a mirror.

If a restroom is provided in the office (and this usually should be the case unless the office is in a larger building with easily accessible public restrooms outside the office), the access to the restroom should be easy from the waiting room, and the restroom should be clearly labeled on or above the door.

Lighting in the reception room should be sufficient for reading and usually is best provided by ceiling overhead light rather than lamps (because lamps can be knocked over or interfere with seating arrangements). Some type of phone access should be provided in the waiting room so that patients can arrange their rides home and other appointments. This phone should either be a pay phone or a restricted dialing local phone, or patients should be allowed access to a restricted dialing phone at the sign-in desk.

Besides chairs in the waiting room, other furniture is not necessary unless you want to use coffee tables with underlying magazine storage racks. Alternatively, wall storage racks for magazines could be used. Magazines should be selected to reflect the tastes and interests of the people who will be using the waiting room. Even if the practice sees only female patients, having some male-interest magazines available in the waiting room would be appreciated by the male spouse or friend who accompanies the patient.

There are a number of considerations in choosing decor for the waiting area. You should decide if you want to have a modern or contemporary decor or more of a cozy, family room atmosphere. In either case, the decor should be consistent throughout the area. If you will have children in the waiting room, it is, of course, best not to have such things as low-level fish tanks, ceramic decorative items, or anything else that would be readily breakable. In general, having artificial plants is a better choice for the waiting area than having real plants, not only because of the easier upkeep (no need for water, fertilizer, or trimming) but also because of the lesser allergy-inducing potential of artificial plants compared to real plants. You may want to provide a television or radio in the waiting room. If a TV is provided, usually a wall-mounted one, high in the corner of the room, can be seen better throughout the room than one on the floor or a low table. A "piped-in" FM radio sound system may be preferable to a radio just set on a table. If a TV is provided and connected to a VCR, you can run continuous patient education or practice promotion tapes on the TV. Recent Federal regulations (which are not being consistently enforced) require an office owner to pay a fee if a commercial radio station is continuously played over the office's speaker system and more than two speakers are used.

In some practices, it may be appropriate to have anatomical models, wall charts or posters, or other educational materials available in the waiting room.

Business office. This area would include the reception desk, paperwork processing area, checkout/billing/cashier area, and usually, the storage area for patient charts and financial records. General guidelines for the size of the business office are that about 125 square feet of floor space is required for the first or main worker and at least 75 (preferably 100) square feet of space for each additional full-time worker.

Probably more important than for any other component of the office, allowance should be made for expansion of the business office area. This area tends to have the greatest concentration or need of equipment (computer terminals, printers, FAX machines, phone systems, typewriters, dictation sets, photocopiers). An important design consideration for the business office is that any portion of it in which confidential patient information is discussed (results of lab tests, call-backs about overdue bills) needs to be soundproofed from the waiting area or other portions of the office in which other patients might overhear confidential information. If the registration desk has a sliding window fronting on the waiting area, then this affords some soundproofing of the conversations behind the desk. Be certain that allowance is made for full opening of cabinet file drawers without interference from other pieces of furniture or doors.

Hallways. The design of hallways in a medical office may seem like a minor consideration, but poor design can result in significant problems in office operation. Building codes may dictate the width of hallways so that they may have to be somewhat wider than might otherwise be planned. One important consideration is that the hallways should be wide enough to allow access by wide-based wheelchairs and/or ambulance stretchers (gurneys) if you may have patients requiring ambulance transport either to or from the office. One fairly easy way to determine if hallways will accommodate ambulance stretchers is to draw the proposed office design onto scaled graph paper, cut out a scaled piece of paper the size of the typical ambulance litter (78 × 22 inches) and maneuver this piece of paper around the graph paper drawing of the office. This makes certain that the litter can be moved into and out of the rooms with clearance of the doors and walls. In general, you should avoid allocating space in the hallways to equipment or furniture because placement of these in a hallway may violate local fire codes.

General guidelines for hall widths follow:

1. A space at least 2 feet wide is needed for a person to walk comfortably between objects.
2. A space at least 4 feet wide is needed for people to be able to walk comfortably past each other.
3. A distance of 5 feet is needed for people to be able to comfortably walk around each other.
4. A width of 6 feet is usually required to maneuver hospital stretchers into and out of adjacent rooms.

Patient examination rooms. The size of the patient examination rooms can vary considerably depending upon the type of patients that are seen and some other factors. If patients will only need to be examined in a sitting position and not necessarily have to fully disrobe for examination, then having very small, almost closet-like, examination rooms may be satisfactory (although closet-like rooms may certainly make patients feel cramped or claustrophobic). Such examination rooms could be as small as 4 × 5 feet. In general, however, most satisfactory examination rooms are between 7 × 9 feet and 9 × 12 feet. Even in pediatric practices, the larger rooms may be necessary to accommodate teenaged patients and the parents accompanying younger patients. In designing the examination rooms, it is important to make sure that whatever type of examination table or bed is to be placed in the room will readily fit through the door.

The basic components of the examination room are listed:

1. A patient examination table, stretcher, or bed
2. Drawer space for equipment storage
3. A small desk or table for the physician to write notes and/or prescriptions
4. A clothing rack or hooks if patients will need to disrobe in the room
5. A sink (optional)

If the office is to have more than one examination room (and especially if a relatively large number of rooms are needed), then you should decide if you want to have identical examination rooms or mirror-image examination rooms. The advantage of having all the rooms "identical" is that the equipment and layout in each room will be exactly the same, making it easier when going from room to room to know where to look for specific items. The construction advantage, however, of the mirror-image examination room is that the plumbing can be located in the same wall between two rooms, thereby reducing the plumbing costs. Again, do not forget to adequately soundproof the patient examination rooms from each other as well as from the hall. This may entail extra wall insulation (more than is needed for just heat conservation) as well as a felt "slider" or weatherproofing strip along the lower and/or upper door edges to lessen sound leak. The presence of carpeting in rooms as well as multiple objects hung on the walls and the use of sound-absorbent ceiling tiles all tend to dampen the sound generated from within the room.

If patients will spend any time waiting in the examination room, consider having magazines or brochures available in the room for the patients to read. This may make their waiting time seem somewhat shorter.

X-ray room. The major consideration with a room dedicated to performing x-rays is to make certain that the room is insulated with appropriate x-ray absorbing material (i.e., lead sheeting) according to radiologic standards. You can obtain the specific construction requirements from any hospital radiology department. One way to get around this structural requirement is to utilize a portable x-ray machine, although the film quality will not be as good. The x-ray room should, of course, also include a dark-room facility (often a separate closet) for a processor and film developer.

Physician's office. In smaller medical offices, a separate physician's office may not be necessary in that the physician could do his or her paperwork in one of the examination rooms. However, having dedicated office space is very helpful to most physicians. The office is probably the most appropriate room to use to discuss prolonged and/or sensitive items with patients. This room would also be the most appropriate place to display diplomas and other items that give the office more of a personal touch. If the remainder of the office complex is not carpeted (because of considerations regarding potential blood exposure or other reasons), it is certainly appropriate to carpet the physician's office not only for appearance but also for further sound dampening.

Staff lounge/meals area. This room may not be considered necessary in smaller offices with a limited number of personnel. However, even in the smaller office, it will appear much more professional to the patients to have the staff take their meals in an area separate from the work area. Generally, the staff lounge should contain a refrigerator (usually an apartment-sized one is sufficient), microwave, and coffee machine. This refrigerator should not be used for medications or lab samples. Either a desk or table should be provided with sufficient chairs for the number of employees that will be using the room at the same time. Whether or not to have a TV in this room depends upon the likelihood that the programs would distract your staff from their work.

Restrooms. For the smaller office, a single small restroom may be all that is necessary. However, in the larger office, especially one in which patients will be generating frequent urine specimens for laboratory analysis, a second restroom for patients within the patient care area will be needed. If patients are in examination gowns, they would appreciate not having to go back to the waiting area to use the restroom. In addition, in larger offices, a separate restroom for the office staff should be provided and clearly marked. If pediatric patients are to be seen in the office, the fixtures in the restroom will need to be adapted so they are usable by small children.

Office laboratory. A 1988 law, the Clinical Laboratory Improvement Amendments, which is just now starting to be enforced, greatly restricts the ability of a private medical practice to operate a medical laboratory. This law defines medical laboratories at several different levels and requires very specific training and supervision of laboratory personnel to be able to perform specific laboratory tests.

The current list of medical laboratory tests that do not require special training or certification beyond that typically employed by existing medical practices include the following tests:

1. Spun microhematocrit
2. Fecal occult blood (hemoccult)
3. Urine pregnancy test (colorometric)
4. Dipstick or tablet reagent urinalysis
5. Urine specific gravity
6. Microscopic examination of urine sediment
7. Microscopic examination of vaginal wet mount
8. Pinworm tape preparation
9. Visual color tests for human luteinizing hormone for ovulation tests
10. Whole blood clotting time
11. Slide card agglutination tests for antistreptolysin O, rheumatoid factor, C-reactive protein, or infectious mononucleosis screen
12. Gram stain
13. Potassium hydroxide preparation of skin scrapings
14. Sickle cell screen
15. Erythrocyte sedimentation rate
16. Whole blood dipstick for serum glucose
17. Semen analysis

This list is currently being debated and may certainly be different by the time this book is published. Even if you do not plan to charge for simple office procedures such as performance of a stool guaiac or dipstick urinalysis, you still need to register your office laboratory with the Health Care Financing Administration (HCFA). Naturally, an annual fee is required. The laboratory registration form can be obtained from Health Care Financing Administration, Attention: CLIA Program, P.O. Box 26687, Baltimore, Maryland 21207–0487; phone 410–966–4280. Because of the current uncertainties regarding how this law will be applied and enforced, including the potential for very large fines being levied by HCFA for noncompliance with the regulations, you may be wise when starting out in practice to limit your initial office laboratory items to those on the "waiver tests" list above. If you want to do tests in the office such as serum electrolytes, coulter counter CBC, liver function tests, or others, you need to meet the specific HCFA requirements for a Level 2 or 3 (depending on the tests) laboratory. To qualify for one of these higher level laboratory designations, the following general requirements must be met.

1. The laboratory personnel must have special training, competence, and certification in performing the tests (this, in most cases, means a degree in medical technology or related equivalent).
2. The laboratory supervisor must have special training, and for certain tests, this in fact mandates having a board-certified pathologist as the laboratory supervisor or director.
3. Specific guidelines for quality control must be met.
4. Inspection of the laboratory by federal personnel could be done at any time and heavy fines levied for noncompliance with the regulations, especially for performance of tests for which the laboratory was not approved. The unfortunate result of the CLIA law has been to greatly restrict the ability to perform laboratory tests in the private medical office. This has led to more practitioners referring their office patients to a hospital laboratory or outside approved medical laboratory for even relatively simple blood work rather than being able to perform these tests in the office. New Federal regulations also mandate that you must formally notify patients of any financial interest you may have in an outside laboratory facility before referring them to that facility, and advise them that they could have the tests done elsewhere instead.

PART 2

Equipment and Supplies Needed in the Office

The following is a list, divided by type of room, for the typical equipment that you would need for your office. Consult Appendix B at the back of the book for a list of representative catalogs from which some of these items may be ordered.

1. Entryway/outside wall
   Entrance/practice title sign
   Open/closed sign
   Outside lighting
   Floor mat
   Doorbell or outside intercom
2. Reception/waiting room
   Chairs
   Coffee table
   Coat and hat rack
   Magazine rack
   Plant stands/containers
   Wastebasket
   Toys/books for children
   Magazines/books for adults
   Television/radio
   Wall signs regarding scheduling/billing/practice philosophy
   Diplomas and certificates
   Drinking fountain or water cooler
3. Business office
   Appointment book
   Calculator
   Chairs for staff
   FAX machine
   Computer and printer
   Filing cabinet/system
   Photocopying machine
   Paging system/intercom box
   Telephone system
   Wastebasket
   Clock
   Dictation/transcription system

4. Hallway
   Wall decorations
   Wheelchairs
   Movable stretchers or carts
   Extra chairs
   Patient chart rack
   X-ray view box
   Fire extinguisher
5. Examination room
   Examination table or stretcher
   Storage cabinets
   Writing table (may be built into a wall or fold-down from wall)
   Movable stool and/or chair for the physician
   Additional chair(s) for family members(s)
   Clothing rack or hooks
   Footstool
   Curtain and track (to pull around to screen the examination table)
   Wastebasket
   Wall chart holder
   Otoscope with bulb insufflator/ophthalmoscope
   Sphygmomanometer (wall-mounted or portable type)
   Mayo instrument stand
   Weighing scales
   Movable overhead lamp or floor surgical lamp
   Bedpan/urinal/emesis basin
   Oxygen outlet
   Suction outlet
   Wall or desk-mounted intercom
   X-ray view box
6. Physician's office
   Large desk
   Several chairs for physician and patients
   Bookcase
   File cabinet
   Plant stand
   Lamp
   Diplomas/certificates
   X-ray view box

Phone and intercom system
Wastebasket
Coat rack or coat closet

7. Staff lounge
   Table or desk
   Several chairs
   Lockers
   Refrigerator
   Microwave
   Coffee machine
   Sink
   "Mail" box for each employee
   Bookshelves
   Wastebasket
   Coat rack
8. X-ray room
   Lead aprons
   Film cassettes and screens
   Developer/fixer solutions
   Developing tank
   Drip tray
   X-ray film (unexposed)
   Film dryer
   Film filing envelopes
   Film markers
   Lead gloves
9. Minor surgery room
   Surgical gowns
   Surgical gloves
   Surgical hats and booties
   Instrument stand
   Kick bucket
   Surgical lamp (either overhead or portable)
   Oxygen equipment
   Suction pump or wall suction
   Scrub sink
   Storage cabinets
   Instrument table
   Crash cart
   Electrosurgical unit

Anesthesia machine
Needle disposal container
X-ray view box

10. Nurses' station
Refrigerator (for medicines and specimens)
Medication cabinet
Lockable narcotics cabinet
Needle (biohazard) disposal container
Storage cabinets
Chart rack
Microscope
Microscope slides
Laboratory equipment (centrifuge and others)
Sample medications
Weighing scale (adult, child, baby)
ECG machine
Sterilizer or autoclave
Blood glucose monitor

PART 3

Small and "Consumable" Items Needed for the Office

The following is a long list of the more minor supplies that need to be considered for use in the office. Obviously, not all specialties will require all of the equipment listed below. Consult Appendix 6.2 for a list of representative catalogs from which some of these items may be ordered.

Patient Care Area Supplies List

Airways oral/nasal
Air splints
Ammonia inhalants
Seizure bite sticks
Rubber tourniquets
2 × 2 gauze
4 × 4 gauze
Gauze rolls
Cotton balls
Triangular bandages

Elastic bandages (Ace wrap)
Adhesive tape
Plaster bandages or fiberglass casting material
Special bandage materials (such as Vaseline gauze and Xeroform)
Eye pads
Syringes (choose TB, 3 cc, 5 cc, 10 cc, 20 cc, 30 cc 60 cc and/or GU)
Hypodermic needles (choose sizes to be stocked)
Nonsterile gloves
Goggles or face shields
Sterile gloves (choose different sizes)
Padded metal finger splints
Stack or frog splints
Knee immobilizers
Crutches
Nonsterile gowns
Sterile gowns
Surgical masks
Surgical drapes/towels
Booties/shoe covers
IV catheters (choose sizes)
IV tubing
IV fluid bags
Splints
Suture trays
Sutures
Steri-strips
Lumbar puncture trays
Other procedure trays
Surgical staplers
Staple removers
Paper towels
Towels
Wash cloths
Tape measures
Silver nitrate sticks
Foley catheters/insertion trays
Irrigation trays
Aerosol nebulizer
Alcohol pads
Antibiotic ointment

Finger ring cutter
Surgical knife handles
Knife blades
Nasal speculum
Bayonet forceps
Diapers
Paper cups
Examination gowns
Extra lab coats/jackets
Paper sheets
Toilet paper
Facial tissue
Sanitary napkins/tampons
Disinfectant solution
Room deodorizing spray
Isopropyl alcohol
Povidone iodine
Distilled water bottles
Normal saline bottles
Vials for medication
Urine/sputum cups
Suction machine (or wall suction apparatus)
Suction catheters
Oxygen masks
Oxygen cannulae
Oxygen tubing
Oxygen tanks
Nitrous oxide tanks
Neurologic hammer/tuning forks
Liquid soap
Head lamp
Shave/preparatory trays
Benzoin swabs/bottles
Surgical scrub brushes
Woods lamp
Eye charts
Flashlight (and batteries)
Anoscopes/sigmoidoscopes
Stethoscopes
Vaginal specula
ECG electrodes

ECG paper
Defibrillator/cardiac arrest cart (and laryngoscopes, endotracheal tubes, emergency drugs)
Camera and film (for photos of patients for medical charts)
Cotton tip applicators
Tongue blades
Bandage scissors
Suture scissors
Forceps
Cast cutter
Fluorescein strips
Heparin vials
Heplock caps
Umbilical tapes
Disposable clamps
Glucometer
Ruler
Pocket mask
Band-Aids
Cast spreaders
Hand lotion
Water-soluble lubricant
Guaiac cards
Guaiac developer
Bed pans
Urinals
Emesis basins
Otoscope specula (pediatric and adult sizes)
Ear curettes
Ear irrigation syringe/catch bucket
Thermometers
Microscope slides (and fixative for Pap smears)
TM agar plates (and incubator) for gonorrhea cultures
Throat/wound culture swabs
Rapid-strep kit

Business Office Supplies List

Alphabetical and numerical dividers for 3 × 5 cards
Alphabetical dividers for files
Announcement cards

Appointment book
Assignment of benefits stamp
Batteries (for clock, calculator, and others)
Business card holders
Business cards
Carbon paper
Cellophane tape and tape dispensers
Check endorsement stamp
Clipboards, legal size
Color codes for files
- Blue Cross
- Blue Shield
- Medicaid
- Medicare
- No insurance
- Private insurance
- Worker's Compensation
- Each HMO/PPO

Computer paper
Copier paper
Correction fluid to match stationery, ledger cards, and insurance forms
Date stamp
Desk calendars/wall calendars
Desk clock/wall clock
Dictionary
Envelopes for announcement cards
Erasers
Facial tissue
FAX paper
File box for business cards
File box for 3 × 5 cards
File folders
Folders for computer printouts
Frames for pictures/diplomas
Hanging folders
Hole puncher
ICD-9 code book, CPT code book
Imprinted envelopes, large #10
Imprinted stationery, (8½ × 11 inches)

Inexpensive #10 envelopes
Label maker (plastic tapes)
Labels for file folders
Labels for hanging folders
Letter openers
Magic markers/highlighter pens
Manila envelopes, 9 × 12 inches
Masking tape
Medical dictionary
Memo pads
Note pads
Padded envelopes (for mailing nonpaper items)
Paper clip holders
Paper clips
Paper towels
Paper weights
Pencil holders and sharpeners
Pencils
Pens (blue, red, black)
Petty cash box
Petty cash receipt book
Phone book
Physicians' name and title stamp
Plain note paper/typing paper
Postage stamps (letter and postcard)
Postal scale
Prescription pads
Printer/typewriter ribbon
Return address stamp
Return appointment cards
Roller, moistener
Rubber bands
Ruled tablets
Rulers
Scissors
Scotch tape
Second sheets for stationery
Self-adhesive note pads
Stamp holder
Stamp pads (blue, red, black)

Staple removers
Staples and staplers
Stickers for kids
Stick-on labels
Telephone/address Rolodex
Telephone message pads with copy
"Thank you" note cards
3 × 5 cards
Three tier file
Thumbtacks (if bulletin board) or magnets (if magnet board)
Wastebaskets and liners
White correction fluid

Appendix 6.1

Sample Office Designs

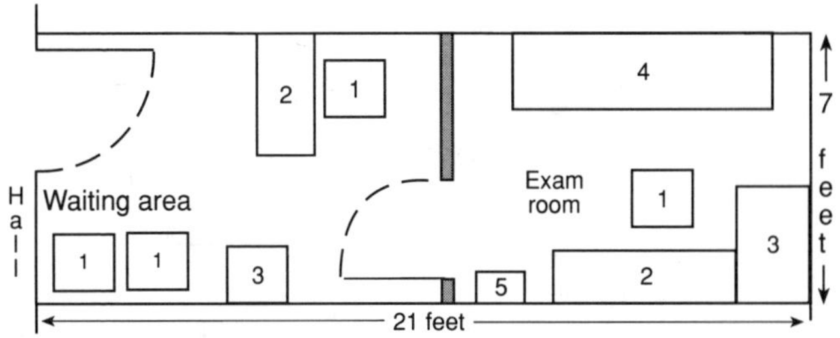

Figure 6.1. The "minimal" or "Spartan" office.

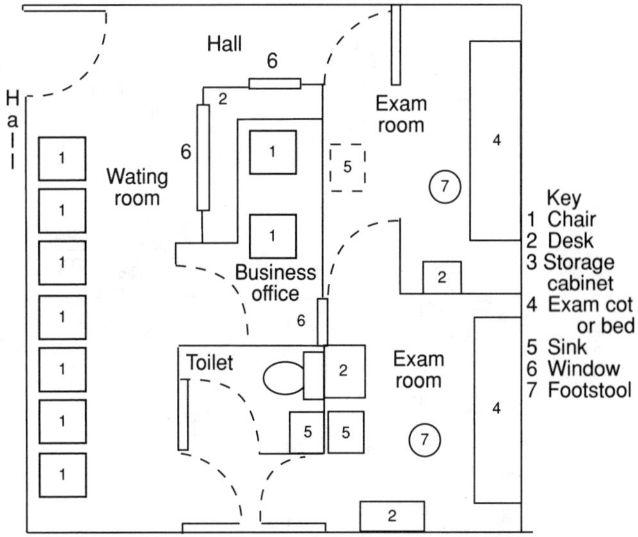

Figure 6.2. The small (20′ × 20′) self-sufficient office.

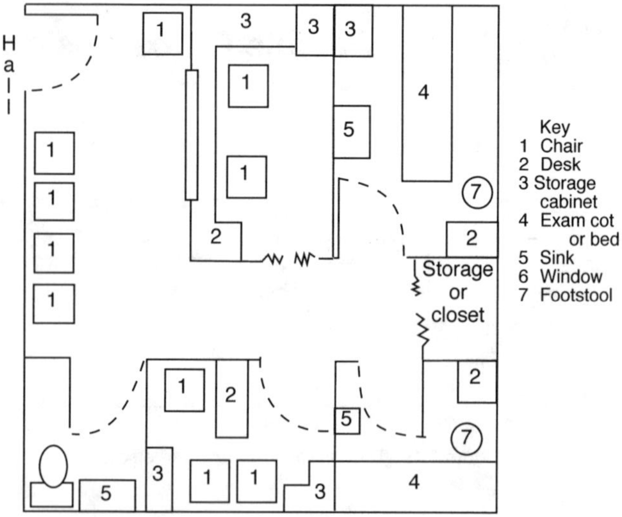

Figure 6.3. Alternative design for the 20′ × 20′ office.

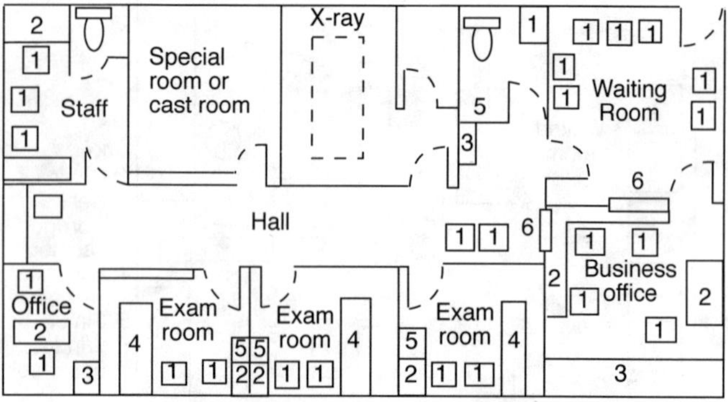

Figure 6.4. Medium-small office (24 by 48 feet).

Chapter 7

Financing and Leasing

GOALS

The goals of this chapter are to present the various options for financing the operation costs of a medical practice.

FINANCING

After having decided upon location and preliminary office design, the next major consideration in starting private practice is the acquisition of financing to start the practice. Financing may be required whether starting a brand new practice, buying an existing practice, or even buying into a group as a new member. If joining an existing group, your contractual agreements with the group may necessitate your acquisition of capital simply to modify or expand the existing office to meet your needs. In general, when starting a practice, financing will be needed for working capital to pay payroll, purchase inventories, purchase new equipment, and pay for office construction. Funds will also be needed to meet your personal living expenses until the practice generates sufficient steady cash flow.

Before talking to a potential lender or financial officer, it is very important to get your financial homework done. This includes preparation of the following paperwork:

1. References from other professionals and/or businesses to establish your credit reliability (as well as credit cards with which you have established accounts)
2. A list of your current financial assets (to include real estate, automobiles, and equipment)
3. A specific list of the equipment, supplies, and other items for which you are requesting money and documents verifying the cost or expense of these items
4. Construction plans, contracts, and formal written estimates from building contractors for your office or office remodeling

5. A formal budget for your office practice, including all anticipated income and expenses and cash flow analyses projected ahead at least several months (this is probably the most difficult item to prepare but is one of the most important items to have available for review by the potential lender)

Construction of your anticipated or projected budget could include the following items:

1. Projected income—This would include average number of patient visits per unit time and the average charge per visit. If you perform a wide variety of procedures or anticipate a wide range of charges that will be billed, you should subdivide this section into the anticipated number of low charge cases and high charge cases. Additional income from interest on any other funds and/or direct payments for other patient care services (such as on-call fees) should be listed and all the anticipated income then totalled over the unit period of time.
2. Expenses—This section should be subdivided:
   A. Payroll—Under payroll, list each employee's salary over the unit period of time and separately list employee payouts for federal withholding tax, social security, health insurance, Worker's Compensation insurance, and others
   B. Malpractice insurance
   C. Property insurance
   D. Other insurance/bonding fees for the employees
   E. Office rent and/or office maintenance fees
   F. Office cleaning fees
   G. Property taxes
   H. State/local taxes
   I. Telephone
   J. Utilities
   K. Equipment rental fees
   L. New/replacement medical supplies
   M. New/replacement office supplies
   N. Journals/subscriptions/medical dues
   O. Pharmaceuticals
   P. Travel/vehicle fees
   Q. Annual license renewal fees
   R. Other

In preparing your budget, you need to account for potential employee payroll/benefit increases, depending upon the length of time over which you project the budget. In addition, some allowance must be made for tax increases, telephone rate increases, and other increases. This would result in some of the expense items increasing over the budgeted period.

After preparation of all this paperwork, the next step is to start shopping for a loan. Consider the following sources:

1. Commercial banks—These are probably the most commonly utilized source of major capital for physician financing. A number of larger banks have dedicated professional banking divisions that deal directly with physicians and other professionals. General advantages of utilizing larger banks are that they may have more experience dealing with health care situations and with medical professionals, may have a larger range of additional services, and may have more backup financial resources. The disadvantages are that they may require more detailed business planning information from you before considering the loan, and they may require you to maintain a cash account balance at their institution to cover 10–20% of the total loan amount that may be in a noninterest bearing account (which they then use as personal security for the loan).
2. A thrift institution—These include savings and loan associations, credit unions, and mutual funds savings banks. The considerations in utilizing a thrift institution are essentially the same as for a commercial bank.
3. Commercial finance companies—These tend to finance proposals at somewhat greater risk than is typical for banks and thrift institutions. The trade-off is that the interest rates from these companies are very often higher than from banks. A greater degree of collateral to secure the loan may be required by this type of institution.
4. Local hospital—The major consideration here is that new federal legislation, which limits physician referral of cases to an institution in which he or she has a financial interest, makes this type of venture between a hospital and physician much more difficult than it has been in the past. If you arrange any practice financing through a hospital, you

should have the terms of the agreement very carefully reviewed by a lawyer, and probably by a Medicare official as well, to make certain that the terms of the agreement do not violate the referral clauses of the Medicare regulations.

5. Leasing companies—Leasing, which is discussed at greater length in a later portion of this chapter, can sometimes be utilized when loans cannot be secured through banks or thrift institutions. Often, the net amount of interest paid over the course of the lease is much higher than that paid on a loan from a bank or thrift institution. The advantage to leasing is that it often allows greater flexibility and convenience in terms of initial and even subsequent payments by the physician.
6. Internal funds from within a large practice—Larger group practices may generate enough internal funds that you could, by arrangement with the practice, borrow money directly from the group to utilize for start-up costs for your portion of the group practice. The total amount of money that may be available by this route may be much less than would be available through a bank, but the repayment terms very often are much better.

In shopping for a loan, you should investigate a number of different sources. For each source, ask the loan officer or bank to prepare a detailed breakdown of the payments and payment schedule that will be required for your loan. The loan officer should split out the amount of principal, interest, and insurance payments that will be paid over the life of the loan. You should take these figures and carefully compare them with loan offerings from other institutions. It is surprising how often the payback features of loans vary such that it may be to your advantage to acquire a loan with an initially higher interest rate because of other more favorable repayment terms.

You will need to supply to the lender specific information as to how loan funds will be used, exactly how they will be repaid, and what contingency plans could be utilized to repay the loan given certain major changes in the practice. The lender will calculate the debt service coverage, which is the ratio of annual cash flow to annual debt service (payback) requirements. The debt service coverage is equal to the net income of the practice, after subtracting physician compensation, interest and depreciation, divided by the principal and interest payments of the loan. A debt service coverage equal to 1 means that the practice generates just exactly enough cash to meet the interest and principal payments. Being able to demonstrate a debt service coverage greater than 1, obviously, would significantly increase your chances of having the loan approved significantly because this ratio demonstrates the ability of the practice to repay the loan (given that all the financial assumptions are correct).

Other factors that may be looked at and calculated by the lender are the current ratio, the day cash balance, and the return on equity. The current ratio is the total current assets of the practice divided by the current liabilities. This measures the ability of the practice to have access to cash to pay obligations, and a ratio of 2:1 or better is considered desirable. The day cash balance is a measure of the amount of cash on hand to meet daily expenses. This is the cash generated in a 1-year period divided by the daily operating expenses (which is calculated by total operating expenses divided by the number of working days in the year). Usually, a minimum of 20 days' worth (4 work weeks) day cash balance on hand is recommended.

Some additional features to go over with the potential lender (which may or may not need to be formally included in a written plan) include the following features:

1. Statement of general philosophy of practice goals and objectives
2. Specific "market" area to be served by the practice
3. Listing of potential competitors and other factors that may interfere with the practice
4. Identification of specific "marketing measures" to attract patients and/or other business to the practice

If your initial loan application is rejected by the potential lender, you should contact him or her directly to find out the reasons for the rejection. It may be that some additional information that you already have available would be all that would be required. Because the lending decision is always somewhat subjective, you may certainly have better luck with another lending institution. It may be necessary for you to secure some other additional forms of collateral for the loan such as temporary hospital financial support or guarantee backing, a spouse's salary, backing from other physicians or groups, or guarantees by family members or other professional associates.

Types of Loans

Loan types can basically be broken down into short-term, intermediate-term, and long-term loans. The short-term loan generally requires complete repayment in 1 year or less and would mainly be utilized to obtain working or operating capital. This would cover such needs as employee payroll, supplies, utilities, and smaller items or equipment. A short-term loan may be all that is necessary to start a practice if it is anticipated that the practice income will very quickly increase. Short-term loans tend to have the highest interest rates, and the rates may fluctuate according to the prime rate of interest. The lender may require the borrower to maintain an amount of money equivalent to 10–20% of the loan as a "holding" balance at the lending institution. Short-term loans usually require less collateral (often nothing beyond the "holding" account) than do longer term loans.

Intermediate-term loans generally have a repayment time period of 2–8 years. In determining the period of loan repayment, it is important to structure it so that it takes the same repayment time as the anticipated time of use of the facility or equipment. Intermediate-term loans generally require significant collateral (such as owning valuable equipment) to secure the loan. Interest rates on intermediate-term loans can be arranged either to have a variable rate (tied to the bank's prime rate of interest, i.e., the rate of interest that the bank itself is charged by larger financial institutions to receive funds) or a fixed rate. Generally, the fixed rate is set higher than the initial variable rate but, of course, has the advantage that the payment amount will be known and constant. Use of a variable rate, however, can be made less risky for the borrower by preestablishing a cap above which the rate may not be increased.

Long-term loans (5–30 years in repayment length) usually are used to finance the purchase of a building or other expensive asset for the practice. Instead of utilizing equipment as collateral, other real estate may often be required as collateral to obtain this type of loan. Some long-term loans are termed "balloon loans," which means they require a "balloon payment" or final payment on the loan that is greater than the preceding installment payments. This final balloon payment finishes paying off the loan in full. Long-term loans tend to have lower interest rates, but the net amount of money paid by the borrower will be much higher over the long run because of the greater number of payments.

LEASING

The previous discussion on loans generally pertains to money obtained to purchase a building or practice outright. The major alternative method of financing involves leasing. Leasing provides the following advantages:

1. Most leasing payments are 100% deductible for tax purposes.
2. If your long-range plans are unclear or uncertain, leasing allows greater flexibility in being able to withdraw without commitment of further financial resources.
3. Leasing usually is essentially equivalent to 100% financing and does not require down payments as outright purchases often do. This allows preservation of working capital and cash on hand for the practice.
4. Leasing allows you to "test out" a piece of equipment or a practice and thus somewhat protects you against the risk of the equipment becoming obsolete and without resale value. Some types of equipment, such as telephone and computer equipment that may rapidly become obsolete, are particularly appropriate for leasing arrangements.

Important Terminology

1. *Gross lease*—This type of lease payment includes all expenses such as operating expenses, utilities, maintenance, cleaning and taxes.
2. *Net lease*—This is a lease payment for the space or equipment only and does not include other expenses. You would probably be billed separately for these other expenses. Net leases are also sometimes referred to as "triple net," meaning that no other payments or coverage are included in the rent fee.
3. *Lessor* is the granter of the lease or the landlord.
4. *Lessee* is the rent payer or tenant.

5. *Raw space* refers to the space in a newly constructed building without inside walls, wiring, plumbing or fixtures.
6. *Turn-key space* refers to the amount of finished, usable, rentable space and should include an area that already has internal walls, electrical supply, plumbing, telephone wiring, finished floor and ceilings, and lighting.
7. *Rentable space*—This represents the sum of the square footage of the area you will actually utilize as well as a portion (share) of the common areas (entrance lobby, public rest rooms, elevators) of the building.
8. *Usable space* then represents the actual square footage that you will occupy and use.
9. *Pass-through expenses*—These are the costs of maintenance, operations, licenses, and taxes on the building. These expenses are "passed through" from the landlord to the tenants. Pass-through expenses can be billed as a lump sum at the end of the year or as an averaged additional payment added to your monthly or other periodic rental fee.
10. *Building standard*—This term should be specifically defined in the lease as to the quality or grades of materials that will be used for particular features of each portion of the building. The portions of the rented space that are visible to the public, such as doors, windows, and entryways, must be constructed of materials that are in accordance with the "building standard." Materials that are more expensive or of higher quality than the building standard can be utilized but not lower quality materials.
11. *Operating lease*—This is essentially the same as a rental agreement and generally covers a period of time that is shorter than that of the useful economic life of whatever is being leased. Operating leases are used for certain kinds of equipment, furniture, cars, and sometimes for expansion office space.
12. *Capital leases*—This term reflects a lease that covers a period of time that is close to the useful economic life of the item which is being leased. The terms of a capital lease often essentially allow the lessee to establish equity in terms of owning the equipment or space being leased.

Once a specific leasing agreement has been drawn up, you should obviously go over it very carefully, and, especially for longer term leases, review by a financial planning officer or attorney is certainly advisable. In reviewing a lease, the following considerations apply:

1. The lease should contain a detailed description of the premises to be leased. This should include room dimensions, all storage space, and any equipment or furnishings (such as carpeting, drapes, lamps) that are provided. There should also be a description of the condition of the equipment and furnishings. The access route to the area should be described, and some type of guarantee that access will not be restricted is often included.
2. Whether the lease is a gross lease or a net lease should be carefully stipulated, i.e., whether the landlord will be paying the utilities, cleaning service, elevator service, landscaping, maintenance, snow removal, minor repairs of furnishings, walls, floors, ceilings, and others.
3. Details of the cleaning arrangements or requirements for the leased space should be given. The specific type of cleaning that will be performed, by whom, and at what times should be spelled out. If there is valuable equipment or items on the premises, it often is advisable to have the cleaning people officially bonded.
4. It should be clearly noted if there is any access restriction or closure of the building after hours, at nights, on weekends, and on holidays. If there is any change in the utilities supplied during these "off" periods, this also should be noted.
5. If you are paying your own utilities, i.e., electricity, water, and others, you should generally have separate meters for these rather than just paying a preapportioned portion of the landlord's total utilities costs. Similarly, you could find out if the air conditioning and/or heating in the building is left on, and to what degree, when no one is utilizing the building, and if you have any control or ability to alter this. Parking arrangements for the building should also be clearly spelled out in the lease. It should be determined if there is restricted or unrestricted access to specific parking spaces and the number of spaces available. If there is any additional payment for parking spaces, this should be clearly noted.

6. The lease should clearly delineate who will pay (lessor or lessee) for improvements in the property, such as replacement of carpeting, addition of built-in desks, and others. If any modifications of the leased space are undertaken, it should be determined if the lease requires the lessee to restore the premises to their original condition when the period of the lease is complete. A "right of first refusal" clause to have an option to rent additional space that might become available in the future adjacent to your allotted space is often a desirable item to include in the lease. Leases should include specific clauses about the ability to potentially renew the lease without renegotiating it. This is referred to as an options clause. For example, having a 5-year lease with two or three 5-year options means that you are initially only making a firm 5-year commitment to the lease but would have the ability to remain in the same space for 15 or 20 years. The options clauses should have specific delineations as to whether the leasing fee or rent may be increased and, if so, by how much. The most common method is to have a clause allowing rent to increase by a percentage equivalent to the consumer price index increase per year, but to define this percentage as a cap beyond which the rent could not be exceeded.
7. Adjustment of the specific periodic rental fees can be done in several different fashions. It may be possible to arrange the initial rent for the first few months of the practice to be lower and then be increased to specific amounts later on, which would allow you greater ease in starting the practice. In longer term leases it may be possible to negotiate to have the first few months be "rent free," which would also allow you to start practice with lesser financial commitment.
8. The lease should specify the exact term of the lease, the beginning and termination dates, and the dates by which options to renew must be signed.
9. If there are any initial separate fees or damage deposits, these should be specified.
10. It is desirable for the lessee to have some type of escape clause in the event of disability, death, or being called to military service.

11. If the lessee will be required to maintain any specific type of liability insurance for accidents to patients visiting the leased space, this would need to be clearly covered.
12. The potential or provision for subleasing or subletting should be spelled out. This could also be allowed for as an "assignment" that would be a signing over of the full lease from the original physician to a completely different physician. (Most leases do not allow for this specific type of assignment but can be readily set up to allow subletting.)
13. It should be spelled out if any of the leasing fees or rent will be credited toward gaining equity or ownership of the leased property; and, if so, if there is any form of a buy-out or balloon payment at the end of the leasing period.

OTHER FINANCING OPTIONS

A completely different route of obtaining practice financing involves the formation of one of the several types of partnership or starting a corporation. A partnership could obviously be established with another physician who would then contribute capital toward starting the practice. However, nonphysician individuals could also be approached about becoming business or investment partners in your practice by providing capital. In this type of partnership, the main considerations would be to draw up a carefully written partnership agreement that would essentially follow the lines of the written contract provisions as detailed in Chapter 5. The contract would obviously need to specify the financial responsibilities of the practice to pay back the investing partner.

In a somewhat similar fashion, another financing option is to form a professional corporation. This represents a form of business organization for a group of professionals joining together in a practice. A professional corporation differs from other types of corporations in that the shareholders of the professional corporation are required to be members of the profession for which it is organized. In this type of corporation, the basic financial structure is that the corporation itself must make payments back to the corporation members (physicians) based on their degree of investment in the corporation. Figuring out whether a corporate structure or a partnership structure is more financially advantageous is very complicated because of the complexity of the current and changing tax laws. In setting up a formal financial partnership or professional corporation, the services of a financial planner and/or attorney will certainly be required because of the complexity involved (which is well beyond the scope of this book).

Chapter 8

Hiring and Managing Your Office Staff

GOALS

The goals of this chapter are to present job descriptions for medical office personnel, review office employee hiring and supervision, and review Occupational Safety and Health Administration (OSHA) regulations on office exposure to infectious materials.

HIRING

When you are just starting in practice it may be possible to have your spouse run the office or business aspects of the practice, or you could even do this yourself. However, under most circumstances, you will not be able to continue this arrangement for very long and still maintain an adequately functioning or sufficiently busy medical practice. At some point early in your practice, therefore, you will need to hire some office personnel. The number and type of personnel needed will depend upon the number and type of patients you will be seeing and on the extent to which you wish to be involved in the day-to-day business aspects of the practice. The most efficient office practices are usually those in which the physician can concentrate on patient care, leaving the management of the business side of the practice to a qualified office manager.

The first thing to do when planning the opening of an office is to decide what initial office personnel will be needed and what their specific duties and functions should be. The major thing to differentiate is whether you will need someone with nursing skills, someone with business and secretarial skills, or someone with skills that overlap these two sets of duties. At this point, careful preparation of job descriptions for the employees you anticipate needing is the best place to start. A job description should include the following elements:

1. Position title
2. Direct supervisor (the person to whom this employee will report and be directly responsible)
3. Job summary (a concise overall summary of the basic duties of the position)
4. List of specific job requirements
5. List of necessary qualifications for the job
6. Salary range and/or benefits (optional)

Positions

There are several positions that may be offered by office practices.

Patient Care

1. Registered nurses
2. Licensed practical nurses
3. Nurse clinicians (Certified Registered Nurse Practitioners)
4. Physician assistants
5. Emergency medical technicians or paramedics
6. Other hired subsidiary or partner physicians
7. X-ray technician (sometimes this function can be performed by appropriately trained and certified nurses)
8. Laboratory technician (sometimes this function can be performed by appropriately trained and certified nurses)

Administration and Business Personnel

1. Office manager—this type of position may not be necessary in a smaller practice but is certainly useful in a practice employing a large number of people who would need to have their activities directed
2. Clinical medical assistant— many of the duties of this type of position could be taken care of by the patient care personnel listed above
3. Administrative (or business) medical assistant—in a smaller practice, a single person could perform all the business functions, whereas in a larger practice, several people with this same title would be necessary to handle the large volume of patient paperwork and processing

4. Insurance secretary
5. Transcriptionist
6. File clerk

SAMPLE JOB DESCRIPTIONS

Job Description 1

POSITION: Office Nurse
RESPONSIBLE TO: Physician
JOB SUMMARY: Assist physician with patient examination and treatment, and coordinate discharge planning and follow-up care for the patients.
SPECIFIC REQUIREMENTS:

1. Bring patients from the waiting room to the examination rooms and assist them as necessary with disrobing and gowning for physician examination.
2. Obtain urine, sputum, and blood samples as requested by the physician.
3. Routinely take and record the patient's vital signs to include height, weight, temperature, blood pressure, pulse, and respirations (as appropriate).
4. Perform ECGs as ordered by the physician.
5. Assist the physician in performance of physical and pelvic examinations.
6. Administer PO, IM, and IV medications as directed by the physician.
7. Open suture trays and minor surgery trays for the physician and assist with surgical procedures.
8. Cleanse and resterilize instrument trays.
9. Assist the patient with redressing, direct them to the discharge billing window, and assist the patient with getting into a car if necessary.
10. Perform appropriate patient discharge education and verify that the patients understand the physician's home care instructions.

JOB QUALIFICATIONS: Current state Registered Nurse license

Job Description 2

POSITION: Clinical Medical Assistant
RESPONSIBLE TO: Physician or Registered Nurse
JOB SUMMARY: Assist physician/Registered Nurse with patient

flow in the office. Assist physician and nurse with patient examination and treatment. Assist with maintenance of the patient care area of the office.

SPECIFIC REQUIREMENTS:

1. Maintain neat appearance and cleanliness of the examination rooms with specific additional cleaning duties as required.
2. Restock supplies and maintain inventory in the patient care area.
3. Assist patients to the examination rooms and assist them with disrobing and draping for examination.
4. Record the patient's vital signs (to include height, weight, temperature, blood pressure, pulse, and respirations) on the patient's chart.
5. Assist in collection of urine and sputum specimens.
6. Record pertinent laboratory, x-ray, ECG, and other data on patient charts as directed.
7. Label specimens for laboratory examination.
8. Dispose of contaminated disposable items.
9. Perform other patient care tasks as directed by the physician or Registered Nurse

JOB QUALIFICATIONS: Six months' clinical experience in a medical office or similar health care setting. Graduate of medical assistant course or similar nursing program.

Job Description 3

POSITION: Registration clerk/secretary

RESPONSIBLE TO: Physician/office manager

JOB SUMMARY: Greet entering patients, route incoming phone calls and assist patients with filling out claim forms and other office records.

SPECIFIC REQUIREMENTS:

1. Greet patients as they enter the office, and notify the physician or Registered Nurse if the patient appears acutely ill or for other reason might need to be seen urgently.
2. Answer all incoming phone calls and route calls appropriately to the other members of the office.
3. Assist patients as necessary in filling out their office medical records and billing claim forms.

4. At the conclusion of the patient's office visit, verify that billing forms are properly filled out.
5. Check messages recorded on the telephone answering machine upon opening the office (and after mid-day breaks if the office has been closed), and post notes about all calls for the physician, office manager, or other appropriate personnel.
6. Assist the office manager and administrative medical assistant with filing and other tasks as directed by the office manager.

JOB QUALIFICATIONS: High school graduate with good communications/interpersonal skills who is able to make patients feel welcome in the office.

Job Description 4

POSITION: Administrative medical assistant
RESPONSIBLE TO: Physician/office manager
JOB SUMMARY: Maintain office scheduling and processing of billing forms.
SPECIFIC REQUIREMENTS:

1. Maintain the patient scheduling book, make new patient appointments and change patient appointment times as necessary.
2. Open and sort the mail, and clip any incoming laboratory or other medical test results to the outside of the patient's chart for physician review.
3. Keep an accurate record of daily charges and receipts and the charge balance at the close of the day.
4. Construct new patient charts and record initial data in the chart; proofread and complete the information recorded by the patient in the chart.
5. Maintain confidentiality of all patient health care data.
6. Gather and verify information for completion of insurance claims.
7. Type reports, correspondence, and dictations as directed by the physician and office manager.
8. Call late or no-show patients and patients behind in payments as directed by the office manager.
9. Maintain inventory of office supplies and forms.
10. Perform other billing and paperwork tasks as directed by the office manager.

JOB QUALIFICATIONS: At least 6 months' business and/or secretarial training beyond high school graduation. Accurate typing at a rate of not less than 40 words per minute. Knowledge of bookkeeping procedures required.

Job Description 5

POSITION: Office manager (note that this job description may need to be more carefully worded than the others in view of the responsibilities inherent to this position; this position needs to be carefully structured so that this person interacts with the physician and allows the physician the relative degree of control and knowledge that he or she wants over the business side of the practice)

RESPONSIBLE TO: Physician

JOB SUMMARY: Overall responsibility for all of the business aspects of the office operation including accounting, billing, and collection of monies. Supervise and delegate tasks to the other nonclinical office personnel.

SPECIFIC REQUIREMENTS:

1. Monitor the recording of charges, receipts, and daily balance by the other office personnel.
2. Prepare monthly summary reports of the office finances for the physician.
3. Conduct regular staff meetings.
4. Interview, assist in selection, train, and supervise all of the business office personnel.
5. Approve credits, refunds, and write-offs in relation to patient accounts.
6. Update or rewrite the office policy manual as directed by the physician.
7. Conduct and update performance reviews for office personnel and terminate office personnel as directed by the physician.
8. Arrange work schedules and vacation time for the office personnel.

JOB QUALIFICATIONS: Master's degree in business administration with some previous medical office or clinic supervisory experience.

Once you have developed a written job description, you should decide upon the salary you wish to offer for the position (this is discussed further later in this chapter).

After determining salaries, you should begin looking for people to fill your office positions. As a graduating resident trying to start a new practice, this can be one of the most difficult propositions in beginning a practice. You may not be able to spend much time interviewing people until after you have completed your residency and arrived in the community. To decrease the time it will take to find a suitable person to hire, try the following steps:

1. Advertise in the local newspapers' classified ads with your practice's specific job description. You do not need to include the exact salary being offered in the advertisement, but if you know that your offer is generous compared to local salaries, then it would certainly be helpful to include it in the advertisement.
2. Check with the local medical society for possible applicants.
3. Contact the American Association of Medical Assistants (One East Wacker Drive, Chicago, IL 60601) for helpful leads.
4. Contact any local business schools or the business department of any local colleges to determine if they have any upcoming graduates or recent graduates who might be interested.
5. Talk with other local physicians and/or the personnel department of the local hospital for leads. However, it is very important not to "steal" a person from either of these sources because it could engender some ill will and interfere with future interactions with these sources.
6. Contacting a local employment agency and/or other personnel agency may be helpful (although often the type of skilled people you may be looking for will not be available through either of these sources).

In your initial contacts or advertisements, you should request that a potential applicant send you a resumé or curriculum vitae. Based on the information in this, you can decide whether or not to pursue the applicant further and contact him or her by phone.

There are quite a number of restrictions on the interview and selection process for potential employees mandated by both the federal government and state governments. In general, of course, it is illegal to discriminate against someone on the basis of race, age, sex, religion, national origin, marital status, plans regarding having children, physical handicaps, and type of military service discharge. The federal government, in fact, even imposes restrictions on the type of questions that job applicants can be asked, and you can be subject to fines or other legal action for violating the regulations regarding potential discrimination. Further information about the specific restrictions regarding interviews and employment application forms can be obtained from the Equal Employment Opportunity Commission of the federal government.

The following is a list of items you might include on an employment application for your office staff. This information certainly could be rearranged in designing your own form.

ITEMS TO INCLUDE IN A STANDARD "APPLICATION FOR EMPLOYMENT FORM"

1. Date
2. Person or source who referred you
3. Name (complete)
4. Social Security Number
5. Present address and phone number
6. Position applied for
7. Date available to start work
8. Education (list high school, college, technical school, and any postgraduate school including the name of the school, address, years of attendance, overall course work, description, and type of diploma or degree)
9. Prior employment experience: name and address of employer's company or business (describe type of company); list all positions for at least the last 3–5 years; dates employed; job title; job duties; starting salary; salary at time of leaving; reason for leaving; name, address, title and phone number of immediate supervisor; permission to contact supervisor as a reference—yes or no
10. Professional memberships or groups (list)
11. Language fluency
12. Specific job skills—for office personnel: typing speed in words per minute, dictaphone transcribing, shorthand, bookkeeping, accounting, computer operations, word processor; for laboratory personnel: specific types of tests which the applicant is capable of performing, certifications; for clinical personnel: venipuncture, starting IV lines, administering IV medications, performing ECG tests, and ability to take x-rays and perform special x-ray procedures

13. Personal references—list name, title, address, phone number, and how many years they have known the applicant
14. Any misdemeanor or felony convictions and give details (except for minor traffic violations)
15. Any physical condition that may limit one's ability to perform the job listed (describe)

Note that questions on national origin, family composition, family planning, religious beliefs, sexual orientation, and other personal items may be in violation of Equal Opportunity Employment Commission regulations and should not be on your employment form. Also, discrimination with regard to employment on the basis of handicaps is prohibited by the Americans with Disabilities Act, passed by Congress in 1992. "Reasonable accommodation" measures are required by the law to allow handicapped persons access to jobs that they might not be able to do otherwise. Exactly how this law will be interpreted and enforced in relation to hiring office staffs is not clear at this time.

After reviewing a sufficient number of employment applications (resumès) and having done some preliminary checking of listed references, you can decide upon which applicants you would like to invite for an interview. At the interview, besides verifying the major pieces of information in the application, you should also clarify any apparent time gaps in the applicant's educational or employment history. To assist the applicant, you should specifically delineate salary and benefits at the interview if this was not already described in your job advertisement or other information that was made available to the applicant. If you are hiring a person who will also be working for a physician partner or will be under another member of the office staff, you should have these other people also interview the applicant. It is surprising how often important information is given or a different impression is conveyed to a second interviewer.

After completing the interview process, you should finish any background checks of the applicant to whom you would like to offer the position. Remember that previous employers may not put down any adverse or negative information about the applicant in written form but may give you considerable negative information over the phone. Once you have settled on the applicant to whom you would like to offer the position, notify this person directly. If the person accepts the position, then be sure to notify the other applicants in a timely fashion that the position was filled. You should thank them and tell them that you will keep their applications on file (generally this is advised for at least 6 months and usually 2–3 years) in case the position reopens.

Because of wide regional variations in pay scales and the unpredictability of inflation, it is not possible in this book to give accurate guidelines for the amount of money you should pay your employees. Probably the best way to decide upon pay scales for your employees is to contact a number of businesses (and/or Chambers of Commerce) in the locality in which you will be practicing. From these businesses you can determine the current minimum wage for employees as well as what businesses of similar size to your own are paying their employees. In addition, calling the personnel office of the local hospital(s) will give you a range of salaries for both medical and business personnel. You may be able to get by with paying your employees significantly less than do the local hospitals because you may not be requiring the employees to work nights, weekends, or holidays. However, it is only common sense that you will tend to attract higher quality workers with better pay scales than they can obtain for similar positions locally.

EMPLOYEE POLICY MANUAL

Writing a carefully detailed employee policy manual before you start your practice is very important. This will give a clear picture to your employees of the structure of the practice, how they fit into that structure, their duties and responsibilities, their benefits, and the procedures they are to follow in relation to the business and clinical aspects of the practice. A carefully written employee manual can protect you from significant legal involvement with employee-related problems. It is generally advised that you compose and write the manual as if it were a legal contract, but include frequent "disclaimer" statements (pointing out that the manual is only a set of policies and guidelines and is not itself a binding contract). Specific information on exact salaries or hourly compensation does not need to be kept in the employee manual because this will often vary considerably from employee to employee and may be revised at frequent intervals. The employee's salary should be stated in the employee's employment contract. Specific information regarding other benefits, however, is appropriate to detail in the employee policy manual. The following is a list of items to consider including in your employee policy manual. Obviously, you may not need to include all of these, depending on the size and scope of your practice.

1. Purpose of the manual
2. General philosophy of the practice
3. General philosophy of the staff's relationship to patients
4. Dates or time period over which the employee policy manual is in effect
5. Procedure for altering or adding to the employee policy manual (it should be noted whether the physicians(s) require the coapproval of the office manager or other personnel in making changes or additions)
6. Specific job descriptions (utilize the complete job description for each different position in the practice as detailed in the earlier sections of this chapter)
7. Specific work hours or specific hours/days the practice or office is open
8. Whether the practice or office will be open at any other times besides regularly scheduled hours
9. Exact times that employees should report to work
10. Time and duration of lunch break and rest or coffee breaks (include whether the office will be open during these times or if the staff will need to stagger their breaks). Federal law mandates a minimum of a 30-minute lunch break and a 10-minute rest period per 4 hours of work.
11. Whether overtime is to be paid and at what rate, as well as any limits on accumulation of overtime pay
12. Whether there will be any expected work time on weekends, "after hours" shifts, or national holidays
13. The days or dates on which the employees are given their paychecks (specify whether monthly, bimonthly, or biweekly; note that if checks are given biweekly, then the employee will receive 26 checks per year whereas if they are given twice a month, then the employee will receive 24 checks per year)
14. Any alteration in the day paychecks are received if the pay period ends on a weekend, holiday, or the office is closed due to weather conditions, or for any other reason
15. If employees receive pay when assigned to jury duty (if their normal pay is much higher than what they receive from the court for jury duty, many employers will continue to pay them that difference during the time of their assigned jury duty)

16. Any provision for salary advance
17. Specifics of additional benefits to possibly include the following:
    Medical insurance
    Dental insurance
    Life insurance
    Disability insurance
    Pension plan/retirement
    Credit Union
    Professional society dues
    Professional journal subscriptions
    Tuition or fees for meetings or courses
    Parking fees
    Use of office business supplies and/or office medical supplies
    Specifics regarding provision of medical care to employees and their families (and at what fee or cost, if any) by the practice or by the physician
18. Length and definition of any probationary period for employment (a probationary period generally would be 90 days during which the employee could be terminated without the physician having to adhere to all of the other employment safeguards)
19. Who sets the salary
20. At what interval or over what time frame salaries are reviewed and altered
21. Specific number of sick days or sick leave allowed
22. Notification procedure by the employee if taking a sick day or sick leave
23. Specific criteria for receiving bonuses and/or merit increases
24. Whether sick days accumulate from year to year and can be credited toward vacation
25. Criteria for use of a "leave of absence" versus extended sick leave
26. Definition of the criteria for a "personal day" or "personal leave"
27. Specifics of any overlap between personal leave and sick leave and whether these days accumulate from year to year
28. Specific paid holidays
29. Compensation provisions for employees who are required to work on a holiday

30. Specifics regarding length of vacation, accumulation of vacation time, and whether vacation time must be taken at the same time as the physician's vacation (this may be necessary in smaller practices)
31. Method for arranging vacation time (include some system for prioritizing vacation requests based upon seniority in the practice, first request received, or any other)
32. Whether employees may opt to be paid for, rather than take, vacation time
33. Whether there is any overlap between vacation time and time for professional meetings
34. Specific employee duties and procedures upon opening the office in the morning and on closing the office in the evening
35. Details of the expected interaction of office personnel with outside business agencies, such as phone answering services, which deal with the practice
36. Specific methods of handling phone calls to the practice (include methods of dealing with patient calls, calls from other physicians and business-related calls); see the expanded information on this topic later in this chapter
37. Specific rules for attendance and punctuality of the practice staff
38. Procedures to be followed in notifying other members of the staff regarding being late or absent for work
39. Policy on receiving personal phone calls by the practice staff
40. Any specifics of dress code, required uniforms when working, or personal appearance standards
41. Whether smoking is permitted in any section of the office by staff or patients
42. Whether or not coffee and/or snacks are allowed or disallowed in certain areas of the office
43. Procedures for reporting work-related injuries as well as for getting evaluation and treatment for these injuries
44. Whether any staff religious activity or political activity will be allowed in the office (generally both of these should be strictly proscribed from the office)
45. Notification period required when resigning from a position or when having employment terminated
46. Specific times or intervals of employee work performance review and criteria for raises and position advancement

47. Whether there is any severance pay or pay for accumulated vacation time at the time of employment termination
48. Specific criteria for immediate dismissal (this would include such things as theft from the practice, grossly negligent care of a patient, showing up for work obviously under the influence of alcohol or drugs, falsification of patient or financial records)
49. Specific performance criteria to be recorded on the employee evaluation forms
50. Statements of agreement pertaining to the practice staff's understanding of the need for absolute confidentiality of patient medical and billing information (the manual should prohibit the employee from discussing patient medical or billing information in any social setting or in any setting where the information could be overheard by a third person; all written patient information such as charts and billing sheets should be maintained in the office in such a way that third parties cannot see the papers)
51. Procedures for release of medical information to any outside party (generally, this will require documentation of express written consent of the patient to allow release of this information)
52. Procedures for use of the office petty cash fund
53. Specifics of the sequence of procedures done in the office including composition of patient charts, billing procedures, insurance form filing procedures, scheduling appointments, arranging hospital admissions and outpatient or inpatient procedures, collecting fees, chart storage and retrieval
54. Emergency procedures to be followed by the office staff in the event of physician illness, unavailability, major weather problems, and others, as well as the emergency procedures for fire or any natural disaster
55. When staff meetings will be held and who may call special or previously unscheduled staff meetings
56. Items to be regularly reviewed at staff meetings
57. Methods for the staff to formally air grievances
58. Procedures for dealing with pharmaceutical company representatives and other sales representatives who may present to the office
59. Procedures to be followed in dealing with particularly disgruntled patients or other types of nonmedical patient problems

60. Procedures for handling blood and body fluid specimens and spills in the office, as well as required educational materials or sessions for the office staff on self-protection from biohazardous materials; this section will need to be extensive and is mandated by OSHA; basically the Centers for Disease Control (CDC) guidelines on "universal precautions" must be met and the specifics of how the office will comply with these guidelines must be carefully spelled out (see Appendix C at the back of the book for more information on this).

It is very important to have all employees of the practice read the employee policy manual and sign a dated statement verifying that they have read and understood all the provisions in the manual. Any updates or changes in the manual should also be read by each employee and you should have some sort of a form for them to initial or sign that they have reviewed the revisions to the manual. Over the course of your practice, you should at some interval (possibly yearly) review the entire manual and bring up any suggested changes or updates at one of the regular staff meetings so that these can be discussed by the entire staff.

It is important to have regularly scheduled staff meetings to maintain an efficient and (it is hoped) happy practice for everyone on the staff. When starting your practice, you should probably have at least weekly meetings of the entire staff. As the practice matures, less frequent meetings will be needed. These staff meetings should generally be held at a time when patients are not in the office and at such time that all the employees of the practice can be there. It is best to have a written agenda for each meeting ahead of time so that everyone's attention can be focused on specific problems and discussion.

To avoid legal entanglements with firing or terminating employees, it is very important to keep written documentation of any problems with an employee's attitude or performance. Maintenance of an employee file for each employee in the practice is very important. This file should generally be kept locked in your office with access only by the physicians in the practice and perhaps by the office business manager. You may want to develop your own employee evaluation forms. The evaluation form should address the following items:

1. Quality of work performed
2. Quantity of work performed

3. Dependability/reliability
4. Responsibility
5. Cooperation with yourself and other office staff
6. Job knowledge
7. Initiative
8. Leadership
9. Innovation
10. Relationship with and treatment of patients

Each of these items could be assessed using either a numerical or a non-numerical scale. For employees who are not performing satisfactorily or up to your expectations (whose employment may need to be terminated in the future), you should carefully note, either on this form or on a separate employee performance form, the particular problem the employee is having. You should review this with the employee. In addition to noting the problem(s), you should note the time period after which the problem will be reviewed or after which continuation of the problem will result in the employee losing some benefits or being fired. The criteria by which the employee's required improvement in job performance will be measured should be clearly stated both verbally to the employee and in written form for the record. Having a well-documented record of persistent employee problems, despite having been given remedial opportunities, gives you very safe grounds to terminate the employment. It should also be made clear to the employee and documented in the record who will be responsible for evaluating their performance, (that is, whether it will be the physician, the office manager, the other office employees, or others).

CONSIDERATIONS IN FIRING AN EMPLOYEE

There are two basic systems under which an employee can be fired. The first involves "immediate dismissal" for specific major adverse behaviors as detailed in the employee policy manual, such as stealing from the practice or maltreatment of a patient. The second involves inadequate job performance, with notification of the employee of the risk of being fired unless improvement is demonstrated and written verification of this. Once the decision to fire an employee has been made, this should be communicated directly to the employee either by the physician or by the office manager. The best time to do this is late in the day, about 30 minutes before the normal end of the office workday. The specific reasons for termination should be directly communicated to the employee. It is best to have a check ready to pay the employee for his or her time already worked and for any additional severance pay that is the policy of the practice.

It is important to recover from the fired employee any key or pass to the office, parking lot, or other practice properties. Someone should probably directly oversee the fired employee's removal of personal possessions from the office to prevent the deliberate destruction or alteration of office records or equipment. After firing an employee, it is important to notify the other members of the staff or practice as well as the manager or landlord and/or security service for the office practice building. This would prevent the employee from being allowed into the practice site after normal office hours. When dismissing an employee, it is important to clarify the type or content of any recommendation you might give for his or her application to future employers. For a particularly disgruntled employee from whom you anticipate retributive problems, you will need to consider changing your office door locks and computer access codes.

HANDLING INCOMING PHONE CALLS TO THE OFFICE

It is mandatory to have very clear-cut policies for your office staff on how you want incoming phone calls handled. There is tremendous malpractice liability for office staff giving patients any medical advice over the phone without your direct advice or input. In addition, there is some malpractice risk in allowing them to make any sort of assessment over the phone as to when a patient should be scheduled for an office visit should the patient have a new or previously unevaluated problem. A simple way to classify the desired response to different types of calls is by a "code number," according to a list:

1. Interrupt me (the physician) immediately; I will take the call (even if I am examining a patient or on another line).
2. Interrupt me immediately; notify me of the call nature and caller's name and I will tell you what to tell the caller.
3. Take a message from the caller and keep him or her on the line; contact me within 2–3 minutes, and I will give you a message to give the caller.

4. Take a message from the caller and hang up; notify me as soon as I am done with the current patient or phone call, and I will give you a message to return to the caller.
5. Take a message and tell the caller that I will call him or her back during our scheduled time for call returns (such as during the lunch hour).
6. Take a message and tell the caller when to expect my return call (at some time other than our usual scheduled time).
7. Go ahead and handle the call without any input from me.
8. If I am out of the office, have the answering service beep me right away and keep the caller on the line.
9. Take a message from the caller and hang up; have the answering service beep me and I will call the caller back.
10. Take a message from the caller and leave me a note to call the caller back when I return to the office.

You should cross-index each of the above choices or responses for the office staff with the following types of incoming calls (this could be constructed as an easy-to-read grid):

1. Patient with new symptoms or a previously undiagnosed problem
2. Patient with unclear symptoms or unclear duration of symptoms
3. Patient with clear-cut, chronic, nonemergency symptoms
4. Patient with billing questions
5. Patient with previously prescribed medication questions
6. Pharmacist with question regarding a prescription
7. Physician with referral or consult
8. Physician with other business
9. Hospital personnel with question about a patient in the hospital
10. Pharmaceutical company representative
11. Business-related call
12. Family member call
13. Other personal call

You should also have a specific policy regarding how patients' phone requests for prescription refills should be handled. In general, the office staff should not be allowed to renew prescriptions over the phone without consulting you directly. One technique for handling these calls is to attach a note regarding the patient's request to the patient's chart and add this chart to the stack of charts containing new x-ray or laboratory results to be reviewed.

Along with this phone call response system, it is very important to inform all of your office staff who your family members are, as well as any other personal friends from whom you may be receiving phone calls. It should be made clear to the office staff how they should respond to these different types of personal phone calls.

RECORDKEEPING

It is necessary to keep very careful records of the employees' work time and payments. In general, this mass of office paperwork should be kept separated from the patient charts and patient financial records. As an employer, you need to verify that each of your employees has a social security number, is not an illegal alien, and is, in fact, able to work in this country. Employment records for each employee should include baseline information on the employee (birth date, occupation title, date hired) as well as details of the employee's work week and payment schedule. These should include, specifically, when the employee's work week begins in terms of day and hour, the amount of hours worked each day each week, and any additional work responsibilities for the employee. The pay for each employee should be recorded in the employment record on at least a weekly basis along with the actual hours worked.

You need to class your employees as "exempt employees" (administrative, executive, or professional status employees) and "nonexempt employees." Exempt employees do not necessarily have to be paid overtime according to federal work laws if they work more than 40 hours in a week. However, nonexempt employees (this generally includes secretaries, receptionists, clerical personnel, nurses) have to be paid at least 1.5 times their normal wage or given compensatory time off if they work more than 40 hours a week. As the employer, you are responsible for making social security deductions and payments, federal income tax withholding payments, Worker's Compensation insurance payments, and fidelity bond insurance payments. As long as you keep careful employment records of both payments and hours worked, it should be fairly easy for you (and/or your accountant or professional management consultant) to determine the payments that you must make to the IRS and other agencies.

PREVENTING EMBEZZLEMENT IN YOUR PRACTICE

One uncomfortable subject to bring up at this point is setting up some safeguards in your practice to prevent embezzlement by your office staff (see Suggested Readings). The best way to do this is to maintain some involvement and monitoring of the flow of money within your practice rather than leaving all the responsibility for that up to the business office employees. The other major preventive step is to have all of your business employees bonded, which means you are insured by a bond insurance company against the employees embezzling funds from the practice. For an employee to be bonded, a rather extensive background check is done by the bonding company of the employee's previous work history and fiscal responsibility. The bonding enables you to recover money lost due to embezzlement by the employee up to the amount for which the employee is bonded.

General Guidelines to Prevent Embezzlement

1. Review the end of day office finance summary sheet or computer printout finance sheet at least once a week (reviewing this every day, if you have time, is preferable). If you review it once a week or less, be certain to choose different days of the week to do the review.
2. Be fair with your employees, pay them well, and do not flaunt your greater income compared with theirs.
3. Periodically check the deposit slips from the bank with the deposit slips from the day finance sheet or computer daily report.
4. Sign all checks used in the practice yourself, and do not use a stamp to sign checks.
5. Do not take any money from the petty cash fund yourself or allow employees to utilize it for personal expenses.
6. Do not have the same employee who opens the mail post the payments.
7. Have all entering payment checks photocopied by another employee before being recorded and deposited.
8. Do not sign blank checks or have financial records recorded in erasable ink or pencil.

9. Review the voided check file periodically to make sure that the checks are in numerical order and none are missing.
10. Have at least periodic reviews of the practice finances by an outside accountant (who does not have a direct financial interest in the practice).
11. Do not allow employees, even the office manager, to take financial paperwork or accounting work home.
12. Perform periodic spot checks, checking the patient's ledger card against the written super bill for that patient's visit and the corresponding daily financial report for the office.

Chapter 9

Office Scheduling, Paperwork, Billing, and Collecting

GOALS

The goals of this chapter are to list the paperwork forms needed, present systems used for office recordkeeping, and review methods for payment processing and collection.

PATIENT SCHEDULING FOR OFFICE VISITS

There are several different systems for patient scheduling, and your choice of system will obviously depend upon the type of patients you are seeing as well as the average time required to see each patient. If your patient population seen in the office consists mostly of follow-up visits (as for brief wound checks, suture removals, blood pressure rechecks), patients can be scheduled at intervals as frequently as every 5–10 minutes. However, if you are seeing patients requiring more extensive evaluations (such as new primary care histories and physical examinations, work-ups for previously undiagnosed abdominal pain, pelvic examinations), you may need to schedule each of these visits for up to 45–60 minutes. If you are not sure how long your patient evaluations will average, then you should keep a careful record of visit lengths as you begin your practice to serve as a guide for future scheduling policies. As you reevaluate and summarize this experience, you can better determine the amount of time it takes you to deal with different types of patient problems in the office and can readjust your office scheduling on that basis. In most medical practices, physicians are seeing a combination of patient visits that only require a few minutes of evaluation and other visits that require more extensive evaluation. Most physicians who see this mixture of patient types find the "modified wave" system of office scheduling to be the best. This system involves scheduling several patients at the beginning of the hour and then a smaller number of patients at 20–30 minutes after the hour, and only one patient later in the hour. The number of patients scheduled at one time obviously depends upon how many rooms are available. Several examples of this type of modified wave scheduling are shown in Table 9.1 (select the choices based upon the average time spent per patient).

In determining your office scheduling sequence, you can, of course, design your own appointment schedule forms or utilize one of the many different forms that are available from medical supply companies. The date and day of the week should serve as headings for the scheduling form as should the physician's name if scheduling is to be done for more than one physician in the practice simultaneously. Columns should include hour of the day and a number of lines for certain minutes after the hour (either one line every 5–10 minutes or using one line for each allotted patient scheduling slot as on the above listed modified wave sequences). Additional columns should include a column to check off if the patient actually shows up for the appointment, a column for patient's name, a column to designate no shows, late arrivals or work-ins (a work-in is defined as a previously non-scheduled patient who would be allowed into the schedule the same day as he or she calls in), patient's phone number, clinical diagnosis or symptoms, and a final check-off column for any additional laboratory or x-ray work required for the visit. Appointment scheduling forms are most effective if the entire day's schedule can be written onto a single side of a sheet. This allows the appointment secretary and physician to review the entire day's scheduling at a glance. In addition to the patient appointment slots, the sheet should specifically list time slots reserved for the physician to make phone call-backs, other phone consultations, meal breaks, and other specific nonpatient-care duties. It is generally advisable in most practices to not fill the appointment schedule with patients fully ahead of time. This allows you to work in both new patients and patients that need to be seen for new problems or new symptoms. The ability to do this in your practice will obviously engender greater patient satisfaction than if patients are always required to wait a significant

Table 9.1
Modified Wave Scheduling System

Time	No. of New Pts Scheduled
Option 1	
On the hour	1 or 2 extended visits, 1 brief visit
20 min past hour	1 extended visit, 1 brief visit
40 min past hour	1 intermediate visit
This cycle would then repeat each hour	
Option 2	
On the hour	1 extended visit, 3 brief visits
30 min past hour	1 extended visit, 1 brief visit
45 min past hour	1 brief visit
Option 3	
On the hour	2 extended visits
15 min past hour	1 brief visit
30 min past hour	1 extended visit
45 min past hour	1 brief visit
Option 4	
(for a really fast physician or one seeing few time-consuming cases)	
On the hour	1 extended visit, 4 brief visits
20 min past hour	2 or 3 brief visits
40 min past hour	2 or 3 brief visits or 1 brief vist and 1 extended visit

time before being able to schedule a new appointment. In addition, there is less malpractice liability if you are able to see patients sooner that have new or previously unevaluated symptoms when these patients turn out to be more serious than they sound over the phone.

It is important to pick a specific time slot for the physician to be able to make phone call-backs to patients. During this time period, no new patient visits should be scheduled. This time period for call-backs is probably best scheduled late in the morning or around noontime, thus allowing patients contacted at that time and found to require urgent evaluation to come into the office later the same day. An additional call-back time at about 3:30–4:00 p.m. would allow patients needing to be seen the same day to be worked in before the usual office closing time of 5:00–6:00 p.m.

Consideration should also be made, in terms of office scheduling, for the other potential interruptions requiring the physician's attention. For example, you may need to allow at least an hour a day (in addition to early morning or preoffice hospital rounds) to answer phone calls or pages about patients in the hospital. If you are taking care of patients in the Intensive Care Unit, you might also need to reserve an hour a day for unexpected return time to the hospital to do patient care in the ICU. Allowance for this kind of "spacing time" would prevent your office patients from being backed up for long periods of time should you be called back to the hospital or have to answer a lot of time-consuming phone calls about patients in the hospital.

Another important consideration early in your practice is whether you will offer evening office hours. This can be very helpful in quickly building your practice. For people who are employed during the day or in school, having to schedule appointments between 9:00 a.m. and 5:00 p.m. may be quite difficult. Evening office hours would not be necessary every night, and perhaps scheduling such appointments as infrequently as once every other week from 6:00 p.m. to 10:00 or 11:00 p.m. might be sufficient to accommodate employed or in-school patients, depending upon the practice's patient population. If you will be scheduling evening office hours, it will, of course, be important to delineate the office staff's responsibilities for evening work as discussed in Chapter 8.

You will find it helpful to review the next day's list of appointments the afternoon or evening beforehand. Having an updated copy of the daily appointments form in the patient care area where you can refer to it throughout the day is helpful in keeping you on schedule.

PROCEDURES FOR PATIENT REGISTRATION AND SCHEDULING

As part of your employee handbook, you should detail the specific sequence that you want your office staff to follow in registering patients. This would include the following considerations:

1. For new patients, have them fill out your standard office registration form and their medical history (to include prior illnesses, prior surgeries, family medical history, social/occupational history, and current medications). The initial registration form should include: the patient's name, address, phone number (home/work); insurance coverage; birth date; referring doctor, if any; names of relatives or other people to contact in the event of emergency and their phone numbers.
2. For returning or follow-up patients, have the office staff verify that the patient's name, address, phone number, insurance coverage and/or employer have not changed.
3. If any of the above items have changed, be sure that these are newly recorded in the patient's office chart.
4. If you wish to know the patient's current payment or account status with your practice, that information or the latest balance sheet should be included with the chart.
5. The patient chart should be delivered to the patient care area of the office. This needs to be done in such a fashion as to preserve the privacy of the patient's chart from other patients or visitors (i.e., do not leave the charts open on a countertop or open in a wall rack in the hall).

Some additional specifics to consider are the procedures that will need to be done by the office staff for scheduling of office patients for laboratory tests, radiographic studies, outpatient procedures and/or inpatient admissions. At the outset of your practice, you need to determine if the local laboratories, x-ray facilities, referral clinics, and hospitals will accept scheduling of patients from your office personnel or if they require the physician to phone in these requests or appointments directly. Be certain that the person doing the phone-in appointments has access to the patient's name, address, phone number, insurance coverage information (to include policy number and other information), patient's age, diagnosis, specific examinations or procedures to be performed, and the indication(s) for the test or procedure.

SPECIFIC FORMS NEEDED FOR THE OFFICE

1. Patient registration form (discussed previously)
2. Medical history form—This could take two forms; one would

be a box check-off form for the patient to fill out, listing potential medical problems or procedures the patient may have or have had as well as additional space for relevant family medical history and social/occupational history. An alternative is that of a standard history and physical with such headings as: history of present illness, past medical history (including surgeries, medical problems, perinatal factors), current medications, allergies, family history, social/occupational history, current vital signs, physical examination, pertinent laboratory/radiographic study results, impression or problem list, and therapeutic or diagnostic plans. For the medical history form, you might want to use a form very similar to what is being used by the hospital or clinic at which you practice (but do not copy this form directly just in case the hospital has copyrighted its own forms).

3. Patient information forms or booklets—These would be papers, brochures, or booklets that you could compose explaining your practice philosophy, office hours and payment policy of the practice, policy on receiving telephone calls from patients as well as providing some information about your medical specialty, special skills, and educational and practice background. These are discussed further in Chapter 11.
4. Prescription pads—You can design your own prescription pads and have them printed, but a very nice source for prescription pads (which are provided to you free of charge and replaced and reprinted as needed) is from the Triple i Prescription Pads Company. Their address is: The Production Director, Triple i Prescription Pads, Box 4170, Cherry Hill, NJ 08034. Their phone number is 1–800–444–3278. This organization will print your prescriptions in the appropriate format for your state and list your name, title, and address according to your specifications. The prescriptions are supplied in a case of pads that should last for an extended period of time, and renewing the supply is easily done by mailing a reorder card to the company. Some pharmaceutical advertisements are interspersed in the prescription pad (and this is why you do not have to pay for them). Some states require you to have special triplicate prescription forms for DEA-controlled substances. In some states, all prescriptions for con-

trolled substances must be written on these triplicate forms and one of the three copies mailed to the state narcotics control board or the DEA. Depending on the state, you may have to order these directly from the state narcotics bureau or have them made by a commercial printer.

5. Excuse from/return to work or school form—These forms, which could be combined, serve as verification for patients that their injury or illness necessarily affected their work or school schedule or capability. You might want to consider having a separate form that merely states that the patient or family member was seen in the office (this may be required by an employer as verification of time spent on personal office visits or transporting or accompanying family members on office visits).
6. Patient instruction sheets—These obviously would vary quite a bit depending upon the most common diagnoses for which you are seeing patients. The most efficient way to utilize these is to compose them ahead of time and have copies run off either on the computer printer or copier machine so they can be given to patients at the time of discharge from the office. In a related fashion, you might want to give patients who are on multiple medications an instruction sheet specifically listing the names and doses of these medications (this, of course, is very helpful to other physicians who may become involved in the patient's care). Also, you might want to give patients a copy of their ECG if they have baseline electrocardiographic abnormalities.
7. Procedure consent form—You could easily adapt the consent forms being utilized at the clinic or hospital in which you practice. The main sections or items to include are: (a) name of the procedure; (b) the major or most likely risks involved; (c) the risks of not doing the procedure; (d) the options to the procedure, if any; (e) additional requests or refusals, such as specific anesthesia restrictions, potential for additional procedures, taking of photographs, or participation of students or residents; (f) a statement that the patient understands the risks involved and agrees to the procedure.
8. Authorization to release medical information—Before the release of patient medical information to a third party (and under most circumstances even to another physician), the patient must sign this form. If a patient signs the form and

you receive this request for release of patient information to another source, you should directly contact the patient to ascertain the reason for the request (inasmuch as this might be the first indication of an impending malpractice litigation). Most requests are simply for insurance verification of the visit and/or procedures performed. The release of information form should specify exactly what information from the chart is to be released (specific visit dates, laboratory results, or in relation to specific medical problems). Under most circumstances, you do not have to release all the information in the patient's chart for a single authorized request. It is certainly legitimate to bill the patient and/or third party for any copying and mailing costs involved in releasing the information.

9. Assignment of benefits form—For a number of medical insurance programs, an assignment of benefits (i.e., authorization by the patient for his or her insurance carrier to pay the physician directly) is included on the insurance billing form itself. Other insurance programs require a separate form to be signed and on file.
10. Health insurance claim forms—The new Medicare reimbursement regulations have required a new health insurance claim form for all Medicare billing. This specific form (which has to be printed in red ink so that it is scannable by computer optical scanners) is available through the American Medical Association (call 1–800–621–8335 for ordering information or use FAX 1–312–464–5600). Most medical supply firms also can supply this type of insurance claim form. In addition to this standard form, you may need to stock other specific insurance claim forms depending upon your locale and the insurance companies that cover your patients. In addition, HMOs and PPOs may require their own claim forms to be filled out, and you should stock these if you have contracts with HMOs or PPOs.
11. Super bill—This is in some ways the single most important form to be utilized in your practice. Of all the office paperwork, the super bill requires the most attention in construction and design. There are so many considerations to be taken into account that there are actually a number of firms which, for a fee, will design a super bill for your particular practice. The super bill basically consists of a form for each

patient, listing the core demographic data for the patient, his or her insurance policy name and number, and the specific examination and procedure fees (by CPT code number) charged to the patient on the current visit. Generally, the super bill should be a triplicate form with one set to be kept in the office file, one to be given to the patient, and one to be sent to the patient's insurance company. If the patient is required to bill the insurance company himself or herself, then two copies could instead be given to the patient. Specific use of the super bill is discussed in the section under bookkeeping principles.

12. Worker's Compensation report form—For each state, there is usually a specific form utilized for Worker's Compensation cases (any illness or injury that is job related). This form needs to be filled out on all cases that would be covered by Worker's Compensation insurance. For employment-related health problems and injuries, the Worker's Compensation system often takes precedence over patients' coexistent private health insurance in terms of billing coverage.
13. Medicaid insurance form—In most states, a separate claim form is required for the state Medicaid program, although in the future this may be further standardized with acceptance by Medicaid of the standard health insurance forms utilized by Medicare.
14. Paperwork that is needed in relation to your own office employees has been discussed in Chapter 8 and would include employment application forms, employee interview/assessment forms, employee evaluation forms, employee warning/dismissal forms, job description forms, employee policy manual, staff meeting minutes form, phone call instructions form, employee contracts, and employee work/pay record forms.

FILING AND RECORDKEEPING

Probably the easiest system for filing medical records is open-shelf filing, ordered alphabetically according to the patients' last names. An alphabet-based file generally results in easier chart retrieval than a numerical sequence file (sequentially assigning patients a number when they initially enter the practice). The open-shelf filing system is adaptable to several different kinds of filing cabinets. Filing cabinets that have the drawers open from the side of the cabinet rather than from the end make the most efficient use of space.

There are a number of choices as to the specific file folders or holders to use for your system. In general, the file folders should be at least 9 × 12 inches to adequately house the usual 8 1/2 × 11 inch paper that comprises most medical charts. Probably the easiest system to utilize involves folders that have color-coded tabs on one side. The side tab could contain two or three letters of the patient's last name with a unique color having been assigned to each letter of the alphabet. This sequence of the three colors on the tab allows files misplaced or misalphabetized to be easily recognized, because their color sequence will be different than the adjacent charts. Additional tabs could be added to the edge of the file to denote other special aspects such as patients belonging to a different physician in the practice, specific medical diagnoses, drug allergies, or coding by type of insurance coverage.

One of the major decisions in designing your filing system is whether to have patient financial information and medical information kept together in the same chart folder. There is some advantage, of course, in maintaining all of the patient's information together in terms of convenience. However, because there is more flux in the billing information and status than in the medical information, the portion of the chart devoted to billing information will need to be changed and updated much more frequently. If billing information is to be included within the same folder as the medical information, it probably should be clipped to the opposite side of the folder so that it is somewhat physically separate from the medical information.

On the medical side of the chart, the information in each patient's folder should be in the same order. You obviously have quite a bit of choice in terms of how you want to construct or order the information in the chart. A standard grouping would include a face sheet with a list of the patient's medical problems and dates at which the problems are active or resolved, followed by the baseline history and physical and subsequent office/progress notes along with hospital discharge summaries and/or operative reports for any inpatient procedures. Laboratory and x-ray reports would follow, and at the end, would be any copies of correspondence regarding medical and/or referral letters to other physicians about the patient. One important item for you to consider with your filing system is whether you want to have included in the patient's medical chart any sensitive personal information about the patient (family situation, sexual orientation) or whether you would want this information to be kept in a separate patient file in a secure locked area in your office. As long as your office procedures ensure confidentiality in the handling of charts and your office staff follows the standard patient confidentiality protocols, it may not be necessary to have a separate "confidential information" file.

In developing your medical chart system, you need to decide if you are going to hand write all the medical information in your charts or whether you will utilize dictated histories and physical examinations and office notes. In general, dictated notes are preferable because of their greater content and legibility, medical-legal value, and ease of copying. If you use a dictation system, often the best method is to have your dictated notes typed onto large adhesive backed labels that can then be stuck onto the 8 1/2 × 11 inch pages in the patient's chart. This would allow you to make additional handwritten notes as required on the pages in addition to the dictated notes.

Whenever a chart is removed from the office, filing an "out guide" is usually necessary. An out guide is defined as a marker to denote that the chart has been pulled from the file. There are a number of different choices for an out guide. A specially colored folder can be used and a card or piece of paper dropped in the folder with the name of who checked the chart out and when. Alternatively, a color tab, listing when the chart was checked out and by whom, could be attached to the side of the file in the position of the removed chart. In general, the original medical chart should never leave the office, with the exception of when it is subpoenaed directly for a court trial (and, in that case, it should be hand-carried to and from the court by either the physician or an office employee).

A system similar to the out guide method can be used to remove or purge inactive charts from the file. One of the easiest ways to do this is to attach a colored tab, coded by year, to the side of the chart to denote the year that the patient was last seen. The first time that a patient comes back for a visit in a given year the color tab for that year is then attached to the edge of the chart. This system allows easy recognition of charts of patients who have not been seen for several years. Depending on the patient's problem, these charts could either be purged from the file or the patient could be contacted to determine the need for further visits.

You should develop policies for how long you are going to retain patient charts even if the patient file is inactive. Probably, retaining charts for at least 3 years would be a minimum because 3 years is the usual statute of limitations for filing of malpractice suits. An exception to this, however, is for the pediatric patient for whom the statute of limitations does not start until the patient reaches the age of 18. Because of the many unforeseen delays in the American legal system, many physicians believe it is prudent to retain charts for an even longer period (even indefinitely) despite the obvious space and expense requirements involved. One alternative, of course, is to have the inactive charts placed on microfilm, but there is a significant expense connected with this. Microfilming can usually be easily arranged through the local hospital's medical records department.

Remember that your office medical charts are subpoenable documents. You should note things in the patient's office medical record in the same fashion you would in an inpatient hospital chart. Extraneous or derogatory personal comments about the patient have no place in the chart and could very well figure adversely against you in a subsequent legal action, if the chart was subpoenaed and reviewed by an outside party.

Be certain that the patient's name and/or identification numbers are recorded on each page of the chart, in case any page were to become disconnected or removed from the chart itself. When making additions to a patient's file, each note should be dated and initialed or signed. Any errors found should be corrected by simply drawing a line through the entry, writing the correction, and then dating and initialing the correction.

No method of fastening the sheets within the chart itself is completely satisfactory. Two-, three-, or five-ring spiral binders can be used. Although these make it easier to add and delete pages, they are somewhat bulkier than other chart systems and require more storage space. Charts in which metal tabs are threaded through prepunched holes in the chart paper conserve storage space but require the most time and effort to change or replace pages. There are several different multiple clip systems that can be used for charts. These can combine some of the space advantages of the metal tab chart with the ease of paper insertion of the three-ring binder. Their disadvantage is that if the clip becomes loose or breaks, the chart may fall apart and mix up the pages.

If you are using a system that records all of the patient information on a computer, you may simplify and condense your medical information storage system. However, with use of any computer system you should have a backup for information storage so that the entire patient file is not lost if there is a computer malfunction. This would involve either periodic printout of the stored data (and then you have the same paper file storage considerations as for a noncomputer system) or keeping a second set of periodically updated disks in a fireproof storage area.

NONMEDICAL INFORMATION FILING

The other files that are necessary for office practice include one for patient billing information, one for your correspondence, and one for your office personnel records. An additional option is a file for medical information/journal articles. This latter file could be done by subject, by journal, or by sequential date.

The employee personnel file should include the work time/vacation time records, salary reviews, sick leave records, employee benefits records, incident reports, Worker's Compensation reports, and employee work evaluations. This file should be kept locked with access only by the physician and/or the (executive) office manager.

Your correspondence could be listed sequentially by date, or separate correspondence files could be constructed for outgoing letters and letters received. Alternatively, you could file the correspondence alphabetically or chronologically by each different correspondent. This could involve separately labeled files for letters to and from attorneys, financial officers, business associates, and others.

There are a number of considerations in setting up a filing system for the practice's financial records. In general, there should be separate files for accounts receivable (monies owed by patients and/or insurance companies to the practice) and for accounts payable (monies that you or the practice owe to others).

The accounts receivable file is probably best done in alphabetical fashion with a separate folder for each patient. Each folder would include a copy of the super bill for the patients's last visit with updated financial information on the patient's account, as well as any correspondence with the insurance company or patient regarding questions or payment of the last super bill. You may want to have color-coded tabs on the accounts receivable charts to identify the date on which the bill was submitted. This allows easy scanning of the file for potentially delinquent accounts that would require recontacting the patient or insurance company.

Your accounts payable file should have a separate folder for each company or vendor to whom you make payments on a regular basis (such as building landlord, telephone company, water company, and medical supply company). Bills to be paid by the practice should be kept in a file (such as a Roladex type or accordion type) so that they can be easily reviewed to determine which bills will need to be paid soon. You may want to break the incoming bills down into two groups, ones that should be paid on the first of the month and ones that should be paid on the 15th or at some other specific time in the month.

BASICS OF BILLING/FINANCIAL RECORDKEEPING

There are quite a number of computerized billing systems available that can process all of your office billing. The structure of all these systems, however, is essentially similar to the "by hand" system described here. The basic and most common billing system utilized is called "one-write" system because it records financial data on several different forms at the same time. The three main paperwork components of the one-write billing system are the day sheet (a large master sheet on which all of the bills or money owed for a single day's visits and procedures are recorded), ledger cards (which record the money owed on a particular day by the patient), and the super bill, which records the examination and procedure fees owed by the patient for a single day or visit.

The patient ledger card, super bill, and the day sheet should each have an area with identically constructed columns labeled date, professional service (name or code number for the examination or procedures done by the physician), fee (the amount of money owed by the patient for these examinations and/or procedures), payment (the money the patient actually has paid that same day), adjustment (any amount of the fee that the physician wishes to write off or cancel), and new balance (the amount of money that the patient still owes after any payment recorded in the payment column). Usually, these columns (date, professional service, fee, payment, adjustment, new balance) are written across the bottom of the patient's ledger card, across the top left hand corner of the super bill, and comprise the columns on the left side of the day sheet. Use of pressure-sensitive or carbon-backed paper on the ledger card and super bill allows the information in these six columns to be simultaneously recorded on the ledger card, super bill, and day sheet. The procedure to do this is simply to line up the columns of the patient ledger card over the same columns on the patient's super bill, which in turn is over the day sheet. As the date, professional service, fee, payment, adjustment, and new balance are then entered onto the patient ledger card, the information is transferred through to the underlying super bill and day sheet. On the super bill and the day sheet are recorded two additional columns, namely "previous balance" and the patient's name. On the right hand side of the day sheet can then be added some additional columns to break down the professional service fee by type of visit, additional charges for procedures, x-ray, laboratory, pharmacy, and others. On the far right hand side of the day sheet could be located a series of columns to record the payment amount from each patient seen during the day that will be sent to the bank for deposit by the practice. This right hand side of the day sheet can then directly serve as a deposit slip for the money posted to the bank for that day by the practice. In summary then, from left to right across, the day sheet would include the following columns:

1. Patient sequence number (the number, in order, of the patients seen in the office that day)
2. Date
3. Professional service (plus CPT code)
4. Fee
5. Payment
6. Adjustment
7. New balance
8. Previous balance
9. Patient's name/identification number

10. Super bill number (the specific individual number for the super bill for the patient for that day)
11. A series of columns that could be labeled to breakdown the patient's bill, such as office visit, surgical procedure, x-ray, laboratory, pharmacy, or physical therapy
12. The next column would be check or envelope number (this could be the individual number on the check received from the patient that will be sent to the bank for deposit by the practice, or a specific numbered envelope containing cash given as payment by the patient)
13. Paid by check or money order
14. Paid by cash
15. Paid by credit card

Each of the columns on the day sheet in which monetary amounts are recorded should have boxed areas at the bottom of the page for totaling these columns. These column totals should also be listed on the right hand side of the day sheet for the deposit slip portion of the sheet. These totals from each day can be utilized to generate the monthly and yearly accounts receivable (money owed) versus the bank payments deposited.

For all patients seen in the office, their super bill should be (at least temporarily) attached to their medical chart. It is most efficient for you as the physician to check off the type of office visit and/or other procedures or studies performed on the super bill. This can be done by another person in the office, but if you do it yourself, considerable time is saved, and charges are less likely to be missed. Checking off the boxes on the form really requires only minimal physician time, but may require significantly more time if that responsibility is delegated to someone else in the office. The super bill should have a space on it to record the patient's next recommended follow-up visit. When you have checked off the items on the super bill, the patient or office medical assistant can then give the patient's super bill (and/or the medical chart) to the office bookkeeper. The bookkeeper then adds up the charges based on the super bill, schedules the patient's next appointment, and writes that appointment date and time on the super bill. The bookkeeper can then place the patient's ledger card on top of the super bill. The super bill is, in turn, placed on top of the day sheet with the columns aligned and then the date, professional service(s), fee, payment, adjustment, and balance are written in on the ledger card, with this same information then simultaneously being recorded on the super bill and day sheet. The payment received from the patient is then recorded on the right hand side of the day sheet on the area that will be used as the bank deposit slip. The bookkeeper can then check the patient's financial folder to see if there are other unpaid bills that the patient owes from previous visits. If a separate payment is made for these previous charges, this could be done on a new separate super bill. The previous ledger card, new super bill, and day sheet would then have columns aligned and the data recorded for this other payment. To do this, the "professional services" column should have listed either "patient payment" or "insurance payment" and maybe even add in parentheses "for previous visit" or similar phrases to that effect. This same procedure would be followed if the patient came to the office just to pay a previous bill or if a payment was received in the mail. Finally, the bookkeeper should give the patient the bottom copy of the super bill (or the bottom two copies if the patient will be sending the bill to his or her insurance company).

At some later interval (often at the end of the month), all of the ledger cards that have a balance due should be checked and follow-up bills mailed to either the patient or the insurance company. Often a copy of the corresponding ledger card could be sent as a bill or statement. Ledger cards for different members of the same family should contain information on each card as to the name and address of the family member who will be responsible for payments. This allows for simplification of billing and helps prevent sending multiple bills to family members residing at the same address.

At the end of the day, the person in the practice designated to make the bank deposits should copy (or tear off the underlying copy if a two-carbon day sheet is used) the right side of the day sheet, which will then serve as a master deposit slip. This person should double check each of the listed checks, cash payments, and credit card payments to be deposited and then deliver these directly to the bank for deposit. Utilizing a master deposit slip such as this, directly from the day sheet, makes it much more difficult for an office member to embezzle money by depositing an altered bank deposit slip.

IMPROVING FEE COLLECTIONS

To improve your office fee collections, be frank and cooperative with your patients about your fees and your practice's payment expectations. It is usually very helpful to have your specific fee schedule listed for at least the most common examinations and procedures that you do. This could be done either as an information sheet on the wall in the waiting room or available as a leaf-through notebook at the sign-in desk. You should also consider listing your fees or at least your practice's billing procedures, expectations, and financial policies in your patient information booklet or brochure. In most situations, it is important to emphasize to the patients that they themselves are responsible for whatever portions of their medical bill are not covered by insurance. The various prepaid health plans (and, in some circumstances, Medicare and Medicaid programs) may directly prohibit you (in accordance with your presigned agreement with the plan) from billing the patient for anything beyond the standard fee payable by the insurance plan. Your office staff will need to become familiar with the complexity of the different insurance plans with which you will be dealing, especially in relation to how deductible payments by the patient are handled. The office staff should also become familiar with the specifics of what services are not covered by insurance plans (some may not pay for routine physical examinations, eye examinations, prescription eyeglasses, or some kinds of home medical equipment). Because of the complexity and frequently changing requirements of the Medicare system, it might be advisable for you or your office staff to frequently call the local Medicare professional service representative to ensure proper Medicare billing procedure when you are starting out your practice. After you get used to the operational procedures involved, you could then decide whether to register with Medicare as a "participating physician." As a participating physician you are allowed to bill only for the preapproved fee by Medicare. As a nonparticipating physician, you can bill a patient for the entire amount normally charged for the service performed, including the difference between the submitted charge and the lower reimbursement that Medicare will pay for the service rendered by a nonparticipating physician. Although you may be billing for higher amounts as a nonparticipating physician, you may have more difficulty collecting the money from the patient than you would receiving the direct reimbursement from Medicare itself. Also, some Medicare patients might be discouraged from retaining you as their physician if you were a "nonparticipating" physician because your bills to them might be higher than from a "participating" physician.

Whenever possible, it is obviously to your advantage to have the patients pay for visits and procedures at the time these are performed. As part of your office procedure manual, you should develop a policy for dealing with delayed payments and delinquent accounts. In general, a bill not paid by 30 days should be pulled and a reminder statement sent to the patient at that time. You may consider having the office staff contact the patient by phone, but this can be very time-consuming effort. Subsequent billing statements should be sent to the patient at predetermined intervals. It is generally recommended that three or four statements be sent at monthly or bimonthly intervals if payment has not been received.

In making subsequent collection efforts, it is important to make sure your procedures do not violate applicable state laws or the Fair Debt Collection Practice Act. This act specifically prohibits the following:

1. Sending the patient any form of bill on a postcard or with words like "past due" or "overdue bill" on the outside of the envelope (because this could be seen by other persons)
2. Contacting the patient at his or her place of employment in such a fashion as to disrupt the normal workday or work responsibilities (this would include contacting patients at improper or inopportune times, such as late at night)
3. Threatening the patient with having the bill referred to a collection agency unless it is you standard policy to do so at that point in the collection process.

As a general principle, it is important, at some point, to communicate directly with a patient who has an overdue bill to determine the exact cause for nonpayment. It very well may be that the patient is perfectly willing to pay the bill and yet has some legitimate financial or personal reason to delay payment. If you are able to determine this directly from the patient, then you may easily be able to work out some form of reduced payment or structured periodic repayment. It is certainly important to be humane and fair with patients regarding their payment of bills, but at the same time you need to avoid developing a reputation as someone who can be taken advantage of or who ends up secondarily bargaining for payment for services already rendered.

If the bill remains unpaid after sending five billing statements or is overdue past 180 days, it is generally recommended that a final statement be sent and specified as such. This statement should specifically indicate at what point in time the account will be turned over to a credit or collection agency. You should, of course, only turn over bills to a collection agency for which you feel you have exhausted all other alternatives. Once a bill is turned over to a collection agency, your return on the original bill will be 20–50% at best.

Before selecting a collection agency to utilize for your practice, you should check with a number of reference sources. These would include the local Chamber of Commerce, Better Business Bureau, local medical society, and/or local physicians with whom you are familiar. Additional reference sources would be the American Collectors' Association, P.O. Box 35106, Minneapolis, MN 55435 and the Associate Credit Bureaus of America Collection Division, P.O. Box 218300, Houston, TX 77218. Since collecting medical bills may require more tact and understanding than business bills, utilizing a firm experienced with collection of medical bills is preferable. It is generally advised that you utilize a collection agency located locally rather than a more distant or out of state firm.

When you turn an account over to a collection agency, you will need to provide all background data on the account to the agency. You should obviously not disclose any medical information from the patient's chart to the agency, but limit disclosures to relevant billing information and patient address and phone number. Once the collection agency has taken over one of your overdue accounts, you should cease billings from your office to that patient. If the patient subsequently contacts you to discuss the bill, you should refer him or her back to the collection agency. Should you actually collect any money on the account after the collection agency has become involved, you should notify the collection agency as they may be entitled to at least a portion of that collected money. In dealing with most reputable collection agencies, you should not have to sign any type of a contract to utilize their services.

Another option to collect an overdue patient bill is to sue the patient in court for it. This step is very seldom appropriate nor is it worth all the trouble and expense involved. In addition, starting this kind of a suit might engender a malpractice suit from the patient in response. Before undertaking such a suit, you should certainly review the credit and collection laws applicable in your state.

PATIENT RECALLS

In addition to having a watchdog system for overdue patient accounts, you should also have a system to follow-up on "no show" patients or those who cancel their appointments. The first and easiest step is to send them a postcard reminder that they should call the office for a reappointment. For a patient who does not "show" or cancels on two consecutive visits, however, a direct phone call or more extended letter is appropriate to try and determine if there is a specific problem related to the visits. You can bill or charge patients for a "no show" visit, but the ill will that this tends to create is generally not worth the financial gain.

Patients who are repetitively delinquent in their payments, frequent "no shows," or often cancel appointments can be formally discharged from your practice. This should be done by a formal letter sent by registered mail to the patient informing them that they will be dropped from the practice and no longer eligible for elective office visits. You should specify a delayed time frame (usually 1–2 months) to allow the patient time to find another physician or alternative source of health care. Within that 1- to 2-month interval, you should provide necessary follow-up care or visits for the patient so as not to be accused of patient abandonment. You should note in the letter that the patient may have their medical records transferred to another physician but that payment of a fee for office personnel time and copying costs would be required.

It is also necessary to develop a system for patient notification or recall based on laboratory and radiographic reports. Rather than let any of your office business or medical staff determine the importance of various laboratory or x-ray reports in deciding whether a patient will need to be reevaluated, you should determine this yourself. The best system is to have new x-ray or laboratory reports attached to the patient's chart as the reports are received and these charts set aside for your review at a specified time of the day. By so reviewing all incoming reports, you will not make the mistake of overlooking a new or abnormal laboratory or x-ray finding requiring urgent follow-up. Once you have had a chance to review these reports, the charts could be returned to the office staff for the appropriate filing of the report in the chart.

SETTING YOUR FEES

Because of unpredictable inflation and wide regional variations, it is not possible in this book to give explicit guidelines as to the specific fees you should set for your practice. There are a number of sources you can utilize, however, to give you an idea of how to set up your fee schedule. The American Medical Association each year publishes an updated fee profile for physicians, based upon specialty, age, type of practice, and region. A fee profile is available from Medicare offices but is usually about 2 years out of date. The county or state medical society may be able to provide you with a range of fees for practitioners in your area. It would certainly be advisable to call a number of practitioners in your practice area. As long as they are not going to be competitors of yours, they probably would readily supply you with their fee information. Once you have determined the range of the local fee structure in your specialty, you should decide if you are going to set your fees at the high end, in the middle, or at the low end of this fee structure. There are obviously advantages to each of these three approaches. By setting your fees at the low end, you might be able to attract more business from patients who are shopping around for doctors, but at the same time other patients might think you were the cheapest because you are not as good or as experienced as other physicians.

In deciding on your fees, you should base them at least partially on your office and practice expenses. In determining this, you need to figure the product of the average number of patients you see per day times the average fee you generate per patient and compare that to your total office and practice expenses. Obviously, your fees should exceed your expenses if you are going to generate a profit. It is patients' general perception that visits for new problems should be generally billed at higher rates than follow-up visits, even though the amount of physician interaction time for these two types of visits might be the same. For most surgical procedures, the surgeon's fee includes some postoperative visits or care that should not be billed for separately unless unrelated to the surgery or remote from the surgery.

In deciding upon your fees, you need to also decide if you are going to have any discounted fees or other allowances for specific patient groups. This consideration also applies to "professional courtesy," which generally means not charging members of various professional groups (i.e., physicians, clergy) and their family members for your professional services. If these types of patients, however, comprise a significant portion of your practice, you may find that you are losing an inordinate amount of money taking care of them. Because most of these patients do have some form of insurance coverage, it is certainly reasonable to extend professional courtesy to the extent that you will not charge them beyond what their insurance covers. You should also determine whether you are going to give professional discounts or allowances to your office staff and/or hospital coworkers, and be consistent in your application of this policy.

OVERALL FINANCIAL RECORDS

It is very important to have a regular summation of the financial status of the practice. For most small to medium-sized practices, summary financial information should be determined at least monthly with a formal financial report being generated. This should include total charges, total discounts/allowances/professional courtesy, total cash receipts, and other income to the practice (this could include interest on accounts, subletting lease fees, HMO capitation fees). Total practice income should then be summed. Practice expenses should be summed and broken down by building expenses, medical supplies, office supplies, salaries, personnel benefits, taxes, insurance payments, and others. The net profit for the month, then, is the total income minus total expenses. Accounts receivable and outstanding debts should be monitored at least monthly. If the unpaid balance is greater than an amount equal to 1 1/2 or 2 months of fees, this may indicate a problem with the billing system, and it should be reevaluated carefully.

It is very helpful to retain a certified public accountant to help you organize your accounting and bookkeeping system, as well as to review the practice financial status on a yearly basis and perhaps help prepare your tax forms. You should clearly determine what the accountant charges for his or her services before services are rendered, as there is wide variability among accountants with regard to fees.

The basic items that need to be kept track of in your financial system include the following:

1. The day sheets of all charges and receipts for each day of the month, a check of the daily balance of charges and receipts (verifying that the summed daily total of charges, receipts, and subsequent balances are correct).
2. Separate records of charges, receipts, and balances for each patient (you may want to set this up for each household or family rather than by patient; this may prevent you from overbilling a single person who is responsible for paying the bills of other family members).
3. A record of the progression or aging of all accounts receivable (this lists the fees owed to the practice according to the length of time the bills have been due; keeping track of this allows you to follow up on bills before they pass an insurance nonpayment deadline).
4. Records of outstanding or nonpaid claims to third party payers such as commercial health insurance, Medicare, Blue Shield/Blue Cross, Medicaid, and others.
5. Records of all bank deposits for the practice.
6. Records of all payments or dispersements by the practice.
7. Records of all employee payroll information and benefits.
8. Records of the petty cash fund and other separate accounts for the practice.

The CPA will obviously need to review all of these data as part of the yearly financial evaluation of the practice.

When starting your practice, you probably will not be able to afford to computerize all your patient and financial records fully. As your practice develops, however, you may want to go with a fully computerized system. Because of the rapidly changing nature of computer systems and companies, it is not possible to give you definite recommendations as to a particular system to purchase. One useful reference, however, is from the Medical Group Management Association, which publishes a regularly updated book, *Software Vendors for Group Practices*. Their address is 104

Inverness Terrace, East, Englewood, CO 80112–5308 (phone 303–397–7888).

In selecting computer software and hardware for your practice, it makes sense to go with well-established companies and vendors. In addition, you probably should visit practices that have already purchased computer equipment to find out the specifics and potential problems of the systems they have purchased. You should also contact your regional Medicare, Medicaid, and Blue Shield professional service representatives to determine which specific computer programs have been approved by these agencies for electronic transmission of claims and would be compatible with their systems.

Chapter 10

Personal Finances, Insurance, and Taxes

GOAL

The goal of this chapter is to review the basics of personal financial planning and different types of insurance.

INTRODUCTION

If you are like most residents, you look forward eagerly to the day when you begin practice and your income increases by twofold, threefold, or more. You may have delayed major financial commitments such as buying a house or even starting a family while your peers in business careers may have progressed rapidly economically. The suddenly increased income that accompanies starting one's medical career can lead to problems unless the new physician makes a reasonable effort to plan and control his or her personal spending. Remember that, along with the new level of income, you will also have significant new expenses; for example, student loan debts, which are averaging $50,000 per physician today, usually require initiation of the repayment process near the end of residency or at the beginning of clinical practice. Also at this time many physicians marry, start a family, buy a house, or start a new practice. It is important to keep a few simple principles in mind and to prepare yourself for your personal financial management just as you prepare yourself for your professional medical career.

The most important principle is to approach your personal finances as objectively as possible. Many people simply do not take the time to think about their personal finances and plan for future needs; they therefore are constantly playing catch-up. A moderate amount of effort is all that is usually required, but unless you make that effort, you will never be in control of your personal financial situation.

This chapter will cover the basics of personal financial management for a new physician. This is not an extensive review, but it is hoped that it can serve as a guide as you are developing your initial plans for medical practice.

WHEN TO SEEK PROFESSIONAL ADVICE

Physicians are notoriously inept at personal financial management. Insurance salesmen, stockbrokers, and financial planners know this and prey on physicians, especially those just entering practice. Your extensive knowledge of medicine and science does not translate into knowledge of personal financial management. In fact, by virtue of being in school for such a long period of time, physicians cannot help but be relatively naive in the areas of financial management.

Virtually all physicians need at least two consultations with financial professionals each year. The first is with a certified public accountant for tax preparation and planning. Having a professional do your taxes can save you thousands of dollars, not only in tax payments but also in interest fees and penalties should you be audited. Physicians as a group are audited at a much higher rate than the general public. When a CPA has completed your tax return, he must accompany you to an audit and defend your return. Accountants also are current on the latest tax code revisions and can give you some general guidelines about ways to reduce your tax liability. Accountants will generally charge by the hour, and their fees will usually range from $50 to $100 per hour. If you do a reasonable job of keeping records, you will make your accountant's job much easier and, therefore, pay less in fees. As a physician, time is your most valuable resource, and taking the hours necessary to complete your own tax return simply does not usually make good sense.

The second professional that all physicians should know is a financial planner; however, arranging this consultation requires more effort on your part. In contrast to accountants, who have a well-established national standard (certified public accountant), financial planning is a relatively unregulated industry. Many people, including many insurance agents, stockbrokers, and others with a vested interest in your decisions, may call themselves financial planners. Your need for a personal financial planner will vary according to the complexity of your finances and the amount of effort and time you are personally willing to spend in managing your finances. However, even the confirmed do-it-yourselfer should meet with a financial planner at least once every two years or whenever there is a significant change in personal financial conditions. It is important to realize that in this area, as in many others, you get what you pay for. To simply rely on the advice of family, friends, or your insurance agent is to ask for trouble. It is well worth it to pay a financial planner for an hour or two of his professional time to analyze and assist in your personal financial planning. When seeking professional advice, look for someone who has completed a course of study and has the title "certified financial planner" or "chartered financial consultant." This means that the individual has completed a course of study offered by the Association of Financial Planning or the College for Financial Planning. Of course these certifications do not guarantee good advice, but they are the only standard certifications available in this field.

In addition to an accountant and a financial planner, you will have need to interact with other professionals on an at least occasional basis, depending on your personal situation. You may need to consult an attorney to review employment contracts, practice agreements, hospital staff agreements, or real estate transactions with which you may be involved. You will also, of course, need a banker for any mortgages or loans, and you will need one or more insurance agents. Remember that these individuals have specific areas of expertise. You should rely on them for advice in these areas, but do not ask them for advice in areas in which they are not expert. As with most professionals, the personal recommendation of someone you trust is probably the best qualification you should seek. You should not be intimidated, but rather you should look at these individuals as professionals providing a service to you. Do not be afraid to ask about their fees beforehand and also find out if they are familiar with the specific needs of physicians.

BUDGETING AND FINANCIAL PLANNING

It is probably safe to say that nobody enjoys budgeting. It is unfortunate that most people's experience with the term "budget" comes in the context of a limitation or constraint on free spending. A budget is defined simply as a plan for spending money.

Making a budget and, more importantly, sticking to it is simply a method for achieving your financial goals, present and future. The advantages of personal or household budgeting are many and include keeping track of your expenses, simplifying the burden of preparing taxes, meeting all your expenses in a timely fashion (and matching them to income), and anticipating cash flow problems. Making a budget does not necessarily mean limiting your expenses but simply keeping track of them and gaining control.

If you have never budgeted before or have tried it unsuccessfully, now is the time to try again. The steps are simple and are outlined below. No matter how much money you think you will have because of your significant increase in income, you may be shocked to find that your expenses can quickly match or even exceed your new level of income. Setting up a budget is really not very complicated, and the most important ingredient for success is to constantly monitor your budget performance. This can be as simple as a monthly review at the time that you pay most of your bills.

1. List all of your sources of income and all of your expenditures. It is often quite surprising to simply go through your canceled checks, bank statements and credit card statements for a year and find out exactly where your money went. Also, you may be surprised to find out how much money is being spent in the cash category, and you may have to keep a log for a week or a month to see exactly where this money is going. If you use a simple computerized spread sheet, this chore can be quite simple and easy to update. Otherwise, use a ledger book or even a yellow legal pad. Do not forget to search for and write down all of your annual recurring expenses, such as dues, memberships, subscriptions, birthday and anniversary gifts, auto insurance payments, and so forth. Total these up and convert them to a monthly amount and add that as another expense. Do not forget to modify this monthly amount as expenses increase.
2. Go over your list of expenses and income and categorize them. There are many schemes that have been used successfully, or you can devise your own. A common categorization system is to put expenses into either fixed or variable categories. Fixed expenses will be such things as rent or mortgage

payments, property taxes, insurance payments, student loans, or auto payments. Variable expenses would be such things as clothing, electric and phone bills, recreation, dining out, gifts, etc. Once you have an organized list of categorized expenses and income, you have a cash flow statement. The cash flow statement itself should open your eyes if you have not used this before. However, this does not constitute a budget. For that you need to move on.

3. List and perhaps categorize your financial goals: for example, immediate goals, "I want to pay all my bills on time this month"; intermediate goals, "I'd like to save a $1000 for a vacation in the spring"; or long-term goals, "I'd like to save $10,000 as a down payment for a house in two years." List all your goals, no matter how unobtainable they may seem at the present time, and then go through and rank your goals in their order of importance. Once you have a handle on all of your expenses (from your cash flow analysis) you will have a good idea of how much of your money you can allocate to your various other goals. For example, if you find that, after accounting for all of your usual expenses, you have $200 per month in "disposable income," you can then look at your list of financial goals and decide how much of this amount you will allocate to each particular goal.
4. The final step in budgeting is to reassess on a regular basis. The effort that you have put in so far has probably helped you to understand where your money comes from and where it goes. However, without constant reassessment your budget will not be successful. A simple computer spread sheet or a commercially available financial management program can be tremendously helpful for this step as well, but even a simple ledger book with columns for expected and actual expenses will give you the upper hand in managing your personal finances.

In budgeting, it is important to try to account for as many recurring or unexpected expenses as you reasonably can. By setting aside a small amount each month, you will find it much easier to pay for that once-a-year "big ticket" item or expense.

Personal financial planning is a process similar to budgeting but represents a longer-term perspective. Whereas budgeting looks at income and expenses on a month-to-month or year-to-year basis, financial planning looks at your overall savings, spending, and earning power. Here is where you must sit down and again list your financial goals (short-term, medium-term, and long-term) and prioritize them. There is no set formula for this process as each person's goals must be individualized; goals also will change as personal and family circumstances change. For example, a young physician entering practice commonly needs to establish adequate insurance, to begin savings and retirement planning, and also may need to plan for repayment of student loans. Later in a physician's career, investments and estate planning become more important and also planning for one's children's education. The important point is to make a reasonably objective attempt to list what your financial objectives are and to devise a plan to achieve these objectives. Here is where an annual or biannual visit to a professional financial planner may be of help. As with budgeting, a regular program of reassessment is in order with financial planning. However, this can be done at a much lower frequency, i.e., annually or whenever your personal circumstances significantly change. Remember that the overall goal of your personal financial planning is to gain control of your finances, and this is not possible without a reasonably regular effort.

BANKING AND CREDIT

Virtually everyone begins their financial life by opening a savings account at their local bank. This is soon followed in most cases by a checking account and then possibly by establishing credit card accounts. Today's banking industry is undergoing tremendous change, and there are many alternatives, such as money market mutual funds and credit unions, which accomplish many of the same goals. Remember that banks are a business like any other and that there is tremendous competition and variability from bank to bank. Do not be shy about shopping around for a bank that provides the services that you want. One banking innovation, which can be a tremendous time saver for the busy physician, is direct deposit of pay checks and other checks into your banking account. Also, the bank card or cash debit card has become almost a necessity in today's world and has simplified the process not only of shopping but also of traveling inasmuch as you have ready access to your bank account throughout the country.

The area of credit and your personal credit history is often a mystery but it need not be. There are only three major credit bureaus in the country, and they are coming under increasing scrutiny by the public and by the federal government. Unfortunately, these services often have errors in credit reports, and these may adversely affect a credit application you may file. You can request a copy of your credit report from any of the three agencies for a \$10–20 fee. This is a good idea prior to making any major loan applications such as a mortgage. You have the right to appeal any information in your credit file, and simple errors are usually easily corrected. You also can add an explanatory note to any credit problems that are not in error.

The three major credit bureaus used throughout the United States and their addresses are listed below:

1. Transunion Credit Information Company
   444 North Michigan Avenue
   Chicago, IL 60611
2. TRW Information Services
   505 City Parkway, West
   P.O. Box 5450
   Orange, CA 92667
3. Equafax Incorporated
   P.O. Box 4091
   Atlanta, GA 30302

These credit bureaus will send you a copy of your credit rating for a nominal fee, and they will waive the fee if you have been denied credit in the last 30–60 days.

Consumer Reports Books (51 East 42nd Street, New York, NY 10017) and the Consumer Information Catalog (Consumer Information Center, Pueblo, CO 81009) are also good sources of information about credit issues.

Credit cards have proven to be the downfall of many people's financial management. In today's world, a credit card is virtually a necessity. For example, it is difficult to check into a hotel or rent a car without a credit card. The problems come when people use credit cards as an unsecured line of credit to buy things that they cannot afford. The easiest rule of thumb to keep control of your credit cards is to insist that you pay off the full balance each month. By doing so, you will avoid the high interest rates (up to 26%) that many credit cards charge, and you will also avoid the tendency to keep a "running balance." If you are using a credit card to buy things which you cannot pay for within a month's time, you should ask yourself if this is an item that you really need or just want. If it is an item that you really need, then you should go through a re-analysis of your budget and figure out what is the best way to pay for it (by credit or by saving for a few months).

Using credit is not necessarily a bad thing. In fact, it is necessary that you buy some things on credit and pay them off promptly in order to establish a good credit rating. Without a credit rating, you will find it difficult to obtain mortgages or loans. Also, using credit cards instead of cash can simplify the process of keeping track of expenses as these are detailed in a monthly statement issued from the card company. If you use a credit card for professional or business use, this can also simplify the process of tax planning. In fact, if you use a credit card for this on a frequent basis, it may be a good idea to have a separate card used entirely for business.

SAVINGS AND INVESTMENTS

If you are like many people, your idea of saving is opening a passbook savings account at a bank, putting your money in it, and never thinking about it again. Likewise, your idea of an investor is a high-powered, aggressive Wall Street investment banker in a three-piece suit. Unfortunately, neither of these images is an accurate reflection of the typical American investor. You do not have to have millions in order to "play" the stock market, and today there are more investment options open to the small investor than ever before. The important thing is to start early in your career and to keep at it in order to achieve long-term gains.

Your investment and savings strategy will hinge on a number of factors, most importantly, your time horizon and your willingness to accept risk. These two factors are related in that investors with a long-term outlook are often willing to accept a higher degree of risk and thereby achieve higher long-term gains. It is important to realize that virtually all investments and savings plans entail some degree of risk. It is generally true that the more risk an investment involves, the greater the potential for reward and vice versa. Bank savings accounts and certificates of deposit are protected by the FDIC or FSLIC and, therefore, have virtually no risk of loss of principal of these funds. On the other hand, they also carry smaller rates of return than other investments. At the other end of the spectrum are so-called "junk bonds" which have a high rate of default. However, they carry the highest interest rates of any fixed income investment.

Most individual investors are far too conservative. They concentrate only on short-term ups and downs in the market or in interest rates and attempt to compensate for these by shifting their assets between investments or savings vehicles. However, this is not a good approach to take. If you are just starting your practice, you have a long time horizon, and your investment strategy should be looking 20 to 30 years in the future. Temporary ups and downs in the market do not have a significant effect when looked at over a 20-year period. It is helpful to consider the long-term average annual rates of return of various investments to illustrate these principles. Over a period of 10 years or longer, no investment beats the stock market for rates of return. During any 10-year period or longer in the last century, stocks have out-performed all other investment vehicles, averaging approximately 10–12% total return per year. Obviously, there will be years with tremendous ups and years with tremendous downs. Bonds, on the other hand, average in the single digit rates of return. Very safe vehicles, such as certificates of deposit (CDs), money market funds, and treasury bills, average 5–6%. When considering any investment alternative, think about what your rate of return will be after accounting for inflation and taxes. Over the last 50 years, the United States' inflation rate has averaged 4–5% per year. As most physicians are in the highest income tax bracket, you can take another 30% or so off of your rate of return for taxable investment income. Thus, a bank CD or money market yielding 6% may actually mean that you are just keeping up with inflation or even losing ground if inflation is greater than 4% per year.

Today, the individual investor has a myriad of options for even relatively small investments in the mutual fund industry. There are hundreds of mutual funds available, and there is almost certainly one that will meet anyone's investment needs. By investing as little as $500 in a mutual fund, you achieve diversification which would not be possible by buying individual stocks, and you are also gaining the benefit of professional management of your assets. You can find mutual funds which invest in specific industries or sectors of the economy. Alternatively, you can invest in mutual funds that seek to match the overall average stock performance, so-called indexed stock funds (which closely match the overall Dow Jones Industrial Average or Standard and Poor's Stock Average Index). Also, there are bond mutual funds, investing in corporate or government bonds. There are mixed stock and bond mutual funds. There are municipal bond funds which can provide bond income free of state and local taxes, and there are also more speculative precious metals, commodities, and overseas stock and bond mutual funds.

When investing in mutual funds, it is important to look for the management expenses, which by law are listed in the fund's prospectus. Obviously, management of a mutual fund incurs expenses related to buying and selling securities, recordkeeping, advertisement, and so forth. These are reported in a standard format as determined by the Securities and Exchange Commission, and they must be revealed in the fund's prospectus. Some mutual funds have lower management costs yet charge an up-front fee of a certain percentage (called the *load*) either on purchase of shares or on redemption. This also is revealed in the prospectus. There are well-known families of mutual funds which are very large, such as Fidelity and Vanguard. These fund families offer the added advantage of being able to switch between mutual funds over the telephone, and these companies often provide excellent customer service.

Another excellent savings option for the beginning individual investor is U.S. Treasury securities. With our national debt reaching record levels year after year, the treasury is forced to issue bonds of various maturities at prevailing market rates. In so doing, they compete with the pool of available investment capital, and recently these treasury securities have attracted increasing attention as yields on bank CDs and other safe investments have declined. The simplest treasury security is the Series EE Savings Bond which can be purchased for as little as $25 either at your local bank or through your place of employment as a payroll deduction. These bonds yield a market rate of interest which fluctuates but is currently guaranteed to be at least 6% per year when they are held for at least five years. Also the interest on these savings bonds is not taxable when used for certain purposes such as children's education. Other treasury securities, such as treasury bills, notes, and bonds, can be purchased through brokers, banks, or directly from the Treasury through the Federal Reserve Bank system.

No matter what savings and investment options you make, there are several general principles to keep in mind. The first principle is the concept of diversification. No matter how attractive an individual investment may seem, you should always spread your investment dollars across several vehicles, including stocks, mutual funds, bonds, treasury securities, and money market funds. This strategy minimizes the risk of loss of capital during economic downturns, changes in investment rates, changes in interest rates, and in case of bank failures. As mentioned above, one easy way to achieve diversification is by purchasing shares of mutual funds. You can also diversify by spreading investments across a time continuum. That is, some funds are invested in short-term investments and other funds in long-term investments. Still another way to diversify is to spread your investments over various regions of the world. With today's global economy, it is almost as easy to invest money in European or Far Eastern stock markets as it is to invest in the United States' stock market. Diversification is a strategy that should always be kept in mind from your first investment onward.

The other major quality necessary for successful investing is persistence. Most financial advisors suggest allocating a certain amount of money for savings and investment each month before other flexible expenses consume all disposable income. This can be as simple as setting aside $50–100 each month, but it is important to be consistent and do it each month. Many mutual fund companies can arrange through your bank to have automatic investments made on your behalf, and this is a simple and painless way to make sure that you contribute on a regular basis. Being as consistent as this has several advantages. The first is that you take advantage of dollar cost averaging. What this means is that the funds you have allocated buy more shares of a stock or mutual fund when the price is low and fewer when the price is high, so that on average you are buying your shares at reasonably good prices. Over time, dollar cost averaging is a tremendously powerful technique, and it will result in higher long-term returns than investment of a single lump sum. The other major advantage of regular investing is the development of discipline. Few of us have the discipline to take money away from some desired cause and save or invest it. However, by "paying yourself first" your saving will quickly become a habit and will no longer seem to be a sacrifice. Many comparisons have been made between the low savings rate in the United States and the higher savings rate in Japan. While this may be overstated in the current political climate, one needs only to look at the Japanese economy today compared to 45 years ago to see the effects of regular savings and discipline. Even relatively small amounts of money invested regularly and allowed to compound over time can result in very significant amounts of capital.

INSURANCE

For most people, including physicians, insurance of various types is the foundation upon which financial security is built. Unfortunately, most people do not understand insurance and, therefore, either do not have enough or pay too much for what they have. The following is a brief overview of the different types of insurance that you may want to consider in your personal financial planning.

The first general type of insurance is insurance for yourself, i.e., liability insurance, disability insurance, and health insurance. These types of insurance protect you as an individual.

Liability insurance (malpractice insurance) is well-known to most physicians and is a necessity of medical practice. This insurance protects you from financial loss from your actions or omissions as a physician. Medical malpractice claims vary significantly by area of specialization, but it is safe to say that there is hardly a physician in practice who will not face a claim of medical malpractice at least once during his professional career. Often, professional liability coverage is obtained on behalf of the physician by a group or hospital. It may also be purchased by the individual through a medical society. By whatever means it is obtained, you must be familiar with the provisions of the policy and in particular what general type it is.

Malpractice policies are of two general types, occurrence and claims-made. The preferred type is occurrence, which simply means that your liability coverage is in force for any acts or omissions occurring during the year of coverage no matter when the claim is actually filed. Thus, you are covered even if a claim is filed years after the time of the alleged malpractice. On the other hand, claims-made policies cover the physician for a specific period of time after which a "tail" must be purchased to continue coverage for late-filed claims. Claims-made policies are significantly less expensive during the period of coverage, but the tail that must be purchased may cost tens of thousands of dollars. If you are employed by a university, corporation or large multi-specialty provider organization such as an HMO, you may have liability coverage provided by the organization on a self-insurance basis. Be certain that your coverage with an organization like this does include a "tail coverage" feature in case you later leave the organization (otherwise you will have to purchase a "tail coverage" policy which might cost thousands of dollars). You should realize that regardless of the means of coverage (insurance or self-insured situation), you as the potential defendant in a medical malpractice suit will have limited ability to influence your defense. The insurance company or self-insurance entity will be looking out for the minimum financial loss involved. Frequently, cases are settled out of court without going to trial. Depending on the circumstances, you should not be unreasonable in demanding vindication or proof of your innocence. Keep in mind that insurance is simply a way to spread risk among many individuals.

The next most important category of individual insurance protection for a physician is disability insurance. Unlike most businesses, which have capital assets, a medical practice, whether single or group, may have as its only asset the labor of the physician(s). If a physician is injured or becomes ill and cannot work, this can put a tremendous financial strain on the practice. Many people consider disability insurance to be as important as life insurance for physicians, especially since an individual's chances of becoming disabled are greater than his odds of dying from an accident or illness (up to age 50 or so). Disability insurance is designed to replace part of your income if you become unable to work. These policies vary from company to company, and they are also available through professional organizations such as the AMA and specialty groups. The important parameter to be aware of with disability insurance is the initial exclusion period or the time you must be disabled before you receive benefits, which may vary from one to six months. In most cases, disability benefits are tax free; however, you should check this carefully in advance with a knowledgeable accountant or attorney. Although it may increase the expense, you should consider buying a disability policy which has an "own occupation" clause. This means that you are considered disabled if you are not able to perform the duties of your usual occupation or specialty. This may be particularly important for a specialist who does procedures. For example, a surgeon who is injured and loses the ability to operate (but who could still function as another type of physician) could be declared disabled by an "own occupation" clause, and then receive benefits from the policy. Without an "own occupation" clause, a disability insurance company may turn down a claim for benefits, stating that the physician could still work even though not in his chosen specialty.

Today, health insurance can be the most expensive form of insurance. Again, policies vary tremendously from company to company, and frequently a health insurance package is offered by the physician's hospital, group, university, or corporation. It is important to be aware of the limitations and specifics of coverage provided through these insurance plans; for example, you and your family may be restricted in your choice of hospital or physician. Group plans and prepaid health plans are generally less expensive than individual or family health insurance plans. As with disability insurance, look into group coverage through a medical society, hospital, or group if at all possible to provide cost savings. Health insurance plans in which you assume part of the risk of hospitalization by means of paying for the first $250–2500 of hospital costs annually (the "deductible") provide maximal savings. Obviously, your family's overall health is a significant consideration in electing such coverage.

The other major type of insurance, life insurance, is primarily for the protection of others. Life insurance protects your family and others who depend on you for financial support in the event of your death. The subject of life insurance is often quite confusing. Its various forms basically boil down to two types: term insurance, and other types which provide cash value or investment along with life insurance coverage. This second category includes such policies as whole life, universal life, and single premium life. These policies are often sold aggressively by agents because they entail larger commissions than simple term insurance. However, if it is only insurance that you want, term insurance is going to be cheaper in almost all cases.

Term life is the simplest and most easy-to-understand insurance type. You pay premiums, and in exchange the policy pays your beneficiary a sum of money upon your death. For equal amounts of death benefit, term insurance will always be the least expensive form of life insurance. The other forms of life insurance all have a savings or investment component, and therefore, the premiums are higher. Whole life is the most popular and widely sold form of life insurance in the United States. While term life insurance the premiums increase as you get older, whole life premiums generally remain the same throughout your life. However, at each age, whole life premiums are generally higher than for term life insurance, and the difference goes into a variety of savings or investment mechanisms which the beneficiary can tap into (e.g., for college tuition or for a home loan). Many people are sold on whole life insurance because it is a form of enforced savings plan. However, you should be aware that insurance companies vary tremendously in their savings and investment techniques and that, with a little bit of personal attention, anyone could accomplish the same goal by investing a certain amount of their income each month.

Universal life policies are a variation on whole life but are more flexible in their investment techniques and also generally guarantee a minimum interest for the life of the policy. Many universal policies charge load or investment fees similar to mutual funds. Finally, the variable life insurance is a variation of the universal policy in that the policy holder chooses what type of investment vehicle and what type of investment risk he is willing to take.

One of the most debated topics in the subject of life insurance is "how much do I require?" There is no generally applicable rule for this, and you must consider your individual circumstances. Obviously, someone with a large family and a spouse who does not work requires greater insurance coverage than someone whose spouse works and whose children are already in college or on their own. For most people, between three and five times their annual income is adequate, and this can be a starting point from which to calculate your individual needs. Also, take into consideration any outstanding debts (such as a mortgage) and any future obligations you anticipate (such as your children's education). You should be sure to review your insurance status on a regular basis, i.e., at least yearly, and make sure that your coverage amounts have kept up with changes in your income and changes in your needs.

Other types of insurance include mortgage insurance which may be a required policy for the protection of the mortgage company or bank in the event of default. This is usually required for mortgages where your down payment is less than 20% of the sale price. Also generally required by lenders is an adequate homeowner's insurance policy which covers both the lender and the homeowner for losses due to such events as fire, weather damage, vandalism, and theft.

TAXES

Taxes are not only a certainty for most people, but they are often their greatest single expenditure. As noted above, it is strongly suggested that you seek professional tax advice from a tax attorney or accountant. However, even if you rely on professional advice, it is important that you be aware of some of the important tax laws as they apply to physicians. Many of the investments that you may make have important tax implications.

Your status as an employee versus an independent contractor will have important tax implications. If you are an employee of a hospital, corporation or group, you will have income tax withheld and reported to the IRS on a standard W-4 form. On the other hand, if you are an independent contractor, you are viewed by the state and IRS as an independent businessman. Your tax will not be withheld, but you will still owe it, and you may have to pay estimated tax payments on a quarterly (every 3 months) or monthly basis. In addition, you may be liable for self-employment tax over and above standard income tax. Similarly, if you are in private practice, you should be aware that the allowable deductions for business expenses change almost on a yearly basis. As always, it is important to keep careful records for business purposes. It is sometimes useful to have separate credit cards and/or checking accounts that are used only for business purposes. If you use part of your home as an office, there are strict rules governing the deductibility of these expenses. Some of your investment and retirement planning will have important tax implications; for example, if you participate in an employer sponsored 401(k) savings plan or an individual retirement account, money which you invest for retirement will accumulate tax free.

This is only a brief introduction into the area of tax planning. You should seek professional advice for the preparation of your tax returns and for tax planning, especially as the federal government continues to make minor and occasionally major modifications to the tax laws.

Chapter 11

Managed Care, Marketing, and Consultants

GOAL

The goal of this chapter is to provide a description of the operation of managed care plans and provide advice on promotion and marketing of a medical practice.

MANAGED CARE

In the medical marketplace, your practice will be greatly influenced, either directly or indirectly, by the growing presence of managed care. Managed care is a term that generically describes organizations that manage and control access to medical services. Included are Health Maintenance Organizations (HMOs), Preferred Provider Organizations (PPOs), Independent Practice Associations (IPAs), managed indemnity insurance programs, and Exclusive Provider Organizations (EPOs). Currently, there are about 600 managed care organizations in the United States with nearly 40 million enrollees. Some areas of the country have more market penetration by managed care organizations than others. In 1980, only 10 states had 10 or more programs, and only California had more than one million enrollees. Today, in contrast, 21 states have 10 or more managed care organizations, and 11 states have more than one million enrollees. Penetration of managed care programs is much more prevalent in urban and suburban areas than in rural areas. Managed care plans continue to be strongest along the two coasts and in the Great Lakes states and weakest in the South.

Managed care programs are currently in a period of consolidation, down from an overall high of 662 plans to about 600 plans. In 1990, 60% of the plans gained in enrollment, 39% lost, and 1% remained the same. It seems likely that a slow but steady continued growth of managed care organizations will occur. Weaker and smaller plans are consolidating with stronger, larger plans. It is increasingly likely that managed care plans will significantly affect your practice.

Means of Physician Reimbursement

Physician reimbursement within these plans typically occurs by one of three means: capitation, fee-for-service, or salary. Capitation is an amount of money paid per patient to a health care vendor to provide insured/covered services to that person for a specific time period (usually monthly). Payment is received by the provider regardless of whether or not any medical service is provided. Total reimbursement received varies according to the number of patients for whom the physician has provider responsibilities. Fee-for-service reimbursement is payment by the patient or their insurance carrier for cognitive or technical medical services. Payments are made on the basis of medical service units or care rendered. Customary, prevailing and usual, or reasonable service fee schedules are common and vary by region of the country. Typically, health care providers are reimbursed at some discount from the fee schedule because of patient volume. Finally, salaried health professionals receive a specified amount of payment, usually renegotiated annually, regardless of the extent of medical services provided.

Characteristics of Managed Care Plans

There are multiple characteristics that may be shared by managed care plans, although much individual variation exists in the industry. Often, such plans allow only a short period for submission of claims (up to 60 days) and promise prompt payment of these claims to the provider (within 15 to 30 days). Managed care plans often have a "gatekeeper." This may be a registered nurse with physician backup, or a primary care physician who authorizes referrals and distributes the patient load to other physician providers in the particular organization. The referral control aspect is crucial; the plan often is not liable for charges and payments without preauthorized referrals. Preauthorization is also a requirement for outpatient and inpatient procedures and nonemergent admissions. Again, failure to obtain preauthorization, except in an emergency, can result in payment denial. Managed care organizations typically reward health professionals for efficient utilization of services. If the expense for patient services is less than the budgeted capitation or fee-for-service monetary limit and there are unspent hospital services funds, some or all of these unspent monies may be returned as a bonus or incentive to the health care providers. Use of providers is coordinated by referring patients only to a certain panel of specialists; all patient information is forwarded to those providers, eliminating waste and needless test duplication. The use of a limited allowed formulary is often encouraged. Generic drugs and less expensive "bio-equivalent" drugs are encouraged. Many times, favored medical service facilities are utilized (radiology, surgicenters, and urgent care centers) that may not have the most convenient location but have the lowest charge for a specific service or procedure. Health care providers may be subject to semi-annual or annual withholding of a portion of their fees until it is clear that practice costs are within the annual budget. If so, fees are returned and bonuses may apply. If not, individual providers are "at risk" for over-budget spending and withheld funds are not returned to the provider. Finally, there is on-going utilization and computer review of inpatient charts and physician visits, referrals, and testing. There are daily reviews to determine if patients can be discharged to a lower level of care or safely go home for outpatient workup of given medical conditions. Sanctions are imposed if "inefficient" physician medical practice is refractory to reeducation or counseling. Such attention is given to primary care physicians and specialists alike. By use of these methods, managed care plans differ from indemnity plans and seek to control costs by means of coordinated care with ready access by providers to patient care information.

No matter which of the types of managed care entities you examine as you go into practice (solo, group, partnership) and elect to join, there are positive benefits to balance against the negative aspects of managed care practice. Be assured, no matter what area in which you choose to locate, a managed care entity is already there or will be shortly. It is very likely you will receive an offer to affiliate with one or more types of managed health care entities. In general, the main benefits of such a relationship are a guaranteed patient base and prompt fee, salary, or capitation payment, depending upon your arrangement. Physicians already in practice in an area with managed care growth may want to affiliate to protect their existing patient base. This is especially true for specialists who will get no referrals (unless they are the only such specialist in a geographic locale) unless they are a member of the managed care system. Primary care physicians will be listed in the managed care directory and will get direct patient assignments from the HMO. Prompt fee payment will aid current practice cash flow whether in the form of a salary, capitation, or a check for fee-for-service procedures and medical practice. This reimbursement base will pay practice costs and limit the age of accounts receivable.

Among other considerations are a fixed schedule with guaranteed vacation and conference time if you work directly for a managed care entity. Cross-coverage between managed care physicians is common. You could encounter significant difficulty in obtaining cross-coverage for your private practice if you are not a member of a managed care plan and agree to abide by their rules and fee schedule. You may have no choice in the matter of whether to join a managed care plan if you join a practice with existing contractual arrangements. In such cases, you must accept the existing ground rules at least until the next negotiation of the managed care contract. (It's best to renegotiate annually.) Finally, some health care providers elect to join plans because they feel medical care wastes, costs, and inefficiencies are being controlled. Similarly, some providers feel voluntary managed care practice is better than a mandatory socialized medicine system, and this participation will slow or eliminate any required national health plan.

Items for you to consider in staff, group, or independent models of managed care plans are similar in nature and scope. In a staff model managed care plan, you are an employee with no initial investment or capital gains or losses. Have your attorney and financial consultant review the all-important contract under which you will practice. The following is a list of the important questions to answer *before* signing a contract.

1. How do medical staff provide input to the corporate board?
2. Do the medical staff elect the medical director of the plan?
3. Are there elected medical staff representatives to the board?
4. Are the medical staff represented on key committees of the organization?
5. How are grievances handled?

6. Is there a contract clause prohibiting arbitrary changes in the contract by the organization?
7. What is the arrangement for contract renegotiations?
8. What are the provisions for dismissal or resignation?

A group model managed care contract should mirror a staff model contract during the probationary period. Evaluate both the medical group's and the managed care plan's financial viability. Request balance sheets and financial statements up front and have an accountant experienced in such matters render an employment opinion. Get a sense of financial security from several group members. Has there been turmoil and staff turnover because of financial concerns or contractual promises that were not met? If so, use common sense and check out alternative opportunities elsewhere. Is the group totally dependent on the managed care plan it services, or is the group involved in multiple health care provider scenarios such that the failure of one enterprise will not bring down the entire practice? Obviously, diversification is a much better situation.

In an independent model managed care plan, contracts are made with solo or group practices to provide care in their offices. Capitation is the usual payment method preferred. Some such entities routinely withhold up to 20% of payments subject to semi-annual or annual review of the physician's hospital admissions and practice patterns. If there is a favorable patient experience, all withheld funds may come to you. If your utilization of admission and testing, even if through no fault of your own, exceeds a predetermined level, you risk the loss of withheld payments and possible sanctions, including dismissal from the plan. However, resource utilization and concerns about unfavorable financial outcome must not lower physician and community standards of patient care. Malpractice risks and the possibility of plan bankruptcy are two other very real concerns. Do not sign any "hold harmless" clauses. You must be true to yourself and provide adequate care for all patients. The standard of care is a physician responsibility, not something a managed care plan can dictate. As stated before, you must take the time to get an estimate of the plan's financial viability before signing a binding legal contract.

Other specific considerations, when reviewing managed care plans, include personal benefits; size, location, and age of the plan; the quality of the plan's health care personnel; and administrative support for different specialists within the plan. Talk with health care members of different plans about pay ranges, vacation, holidays, sick time, CME time, insurance, and pension plans to get a feel for the scope of the benefit plan and to determine areas for discussion and inclusion in a personal provider contract. Whatever the salary arrangement you negotiate, annual cost of living raises are standard. Carefully seek advice from your attorney on negotiable items such as bonuses, positive and negative incentives for practice performance, and malpractice coverage, particularly any insurance "tail" coverage responsibility you may incur should you leave the practice.

While size is no guarantee of future success or viability, the industry trend has been to consolidate smaller plans to achieve economies of scale and stability of operation. Look for medium to larger size plans. Check health staff turnover times. Be sure the "warm body" attitude, with little more than lip service to health staff concerns, is not a problem. Be sure major plan clients are stable if possible. Investigate before, not after, signing a contract.

In general, consider only plans with seven or more years of operation. Administrative experience is invaluable in the operation and continued success of managed care plans. Carefully seek out health care provider personnel and meet them early in the selection and employment process. Are there similar backgrounds, training, ongoing interests, and common ground for the provision of quality medical care? What is the prevailing corporate culture? Are people happy and actively pursuing their careers or simply waiting to move onward? Do they seem helpful? Are they team players? Is there adequate access to a full team of specialists? Are the ancillary personnel cheerful and happy, or overworked, sullen, and underpaid? Watch the staff work; you will learn volumes by spending a day at the office prior to signing any employment agreement.

Location should be a priority in your own and your significant other's (if any) decision as to where to live and work. The advantages of living in the area of your choice should be weighed against any disadvantages of the workplace. Another consideration is that certain practices may be preferred over others in managed care plans. Subspecialty providers may not be paid nearly as well as in private practice; however, affiliating with a managed care plan may provide a guaranteed income level, more leisure time, and schedule control. You may also have the luxury to practice your specialty exclusively rather mix general medicine with specialty services because of financial considerations.

Health Maintenance Organizations

Having now considered the general characteristics of managed care plans, we move onto specific consideration of each type with emphasis on the positive and negative aspects of each. Health Maintenance Organization (HMO) is a term specifically coined in the HMO Act of 1970 (P.L. 93-222) and its amendments. An HMO is a legally defined organization, either nonprofit or for-profit, established for the provision and delivery of a defined set of comprehensive health maintenance and treatment services to a patient group in a defined geographic area. Patients may be enrolled voluntarily or assigned to the HMO by their employer. Provider payment is prenegotiated and may be based upon capitation, fee-for-service, or salaried arrangement. Approximately 40% of all managed care plans are based upon staff, group, or network HMO models. The first modern HMOs were a farmers' cooperative in the late 1920s in Elk City, Oklahoma and the Roos-Loos Medical Group in Los Angeles, California. Dr. Sidney Garfield organized the Kaiser-Permanente group during the 1920s and 1930s on the West Coast. HMOs have grown, and today, despite individual nuances, share certain basic principles. Patients are enrollees and services are provided through an organized system of health providers. Benefits are comprehensive with little out-of-pocket cost for patients and are financed by a fixed, periodic payment.

In the staff model HMO, physicians (providers) are all salaried by the HMO. The HMO and the physicians (providers) comprise one organization. In the group model, the HMO contracts with a multi-specialty medical group as well as separately with hospitals and specialty services such as psychiatry. In the network model, the HMO contracts with multiple groups, solo physicians, or specialty services. In the group and network models, fee-for-service or capitation agreements are the norm. Obviously, many hybrids of these three basic types exist. Often, the HMO may contract with Independent Practice Associations (IPAs) or Preferred Provider Organizations (PPOs).

The key HMO feature is integration and control of health care financing and delivery. The enrollees are entitled to all covered services for a fixed amount of payment per contractual time period. Prepayment provides a fixed HMO budget and risk-related incentives for efficiency; an organized care system provides the mechanism for fulfilling provider commitments. Enrollees have no claim forms or paperwork to fill out, face lower out-of-pocket costs, and have no worries regarding medical coverage for catastrophic illnesses or accidents. As a point of information, the staff model HMO comprises about 10% of all managed care plans, the group model HMO about 14%, and the network model HMO about 16%.

Independent Practice Associations

The majority of managed care plans (the other 60%) are Independent Practice Associations (IPAs). Physicians remain in private practice, usually fee-for-service, with an agreed-upon fee schedule. The physicians own or join a corporate entity (the IPA) which contracts with a HMO. The IPA is usually capitated by the HMO and there may be several HMOs served by the IPA or several IPAs serving the HMO. This is the most complicated model and the one least preferred by HMOs because of the obvious decrease in direct control by the HMO. IPAs work very much like unions. The IPA provider (physician) may pay a fee to join the IPA or may be a part owner. The IPA manages billing and collection forms to promote timely provider payment from the HMO. There is no direct provider negotiation with the HMO. The IPA negotiates a contract with the HMO, and directly negotiates fee schedules, or capitation charges, provider bonuses, or sharing of excess hospitalization incentive funds. A provider-owned IPA gives its membership a larger voice in the content of the contract with the HMO.

A set amount of money is available to the HMO to finance its medical care obligations to the enrollees. These funds come from such sources as premiums from subscribers and return on investments and must pay for all the HMO's expenses (including hospital care, physician fees, administration, reinsurance, etc.). If the HMO is a for-profit organization, a certain percentage of funds are due to its owners and shareholders. In a not-for-profit HMO, these funds can be used in a variety of ways, such as the purchase of new facilities, equipment, new technology, or health care provider and personnel bonuses or incentives. Re-insurance is a means by which the HMO can limit its per case risk for medical expenditures for individual catastrophic illness or accident cases.

The funds for enrollee care obligations are divided into three cost areas: HMO, IPA, and hospital. Contractual agreements regulate the obligations of each cost area. The IPA and hospital area costs are often called the Net Premium. This is the sum the HMO pays out to all providers. It is important to realize that approximately 70% of all managed care plans are now for-profit entities. HMOs will earnestly try to meet their return on investment obligations to their owners or shareholders. Since funds are fixed, understanding the flow of funds is crucial to providers. An increase in costs in one area must be offset by a cost decrease in another area. Providers, simply put, are at great risk from factors beyond their control; for example, an increase in HMO administrative costs may decrease monies available for provider services.

Evalauating Contracts with Managed Care Plans

In the next section, we will explore what you, as a physician provider, should watch out for when evaluating (and before signing) a contract with any managed care entity.

First and foremost, before you actually negotiate or sign a contract, assemble your own team of advisors. This team should include a seasoned contract attorney (who has represented physicians in similar situations in the geographic area at least several times before), a financial planner, an insurance agent, and a certified public accountant. All these advisors should be experienced in dealing with health care providers. Be sure the advisors have no hidden biases against health care providers as a group. Seek suggestions and references from colleagues, the medical society, the bar association, and other appropriate professional organizations. If you do not like the team you put on the field, you are the coach! Change the lineup until you are comfortable and are realizing results that justify your effort and expense.

Next, take the time to assemble the following information about the organizations in which you are genuinely interested. The following checklist contains pertinent corporate background information you can clarify during the interview process. You and your support team must know this information to negotiate a final contract.

Clarify these questions before joining a managed care organization:

1. How long has the organization been in business?
2. How many patients are enrolled and from what geographic areas are they drawn?
3. What employers or businesses are contracted with the organization?
4. What other employers or patients are targeted by marketing efforts to join the plan?
5. Who are the executives running the organization?
6. What is the proof of the financial stability of the organization?
7. What physicians belong to the organization or are contracted with the plan?
8. What hospitals and other health care facilities are contracted with the plan?
9. How will patients be referred to you?
10. Is there a fee to join or maintain membership?
11. How will you be paid? (capitation, fee schedule, etc.)
12. Is a percentage of fees or capitation withheld for administrative costs?
13. How often and by what specific mechanism will you be paid?
14. Is there risk sharing by the enrolled providers?
15. How is quality of service assessed and controlled?
16. Can you send patients to other specialists or facilities?
17. Must you utilize a specific laboratory or other support service?
18. What are the arrangements for malpractice insurance?
19. What office paperwork is required?
20. Are there copayments by patients and are there limits or adjustments to these?
21. What are the mechanisms to void or withdraw from the contract?
22. Has a state or specialty medical association written an analysis of the organization?

The contract itself is a legally binding written instrument between two or more parties who have reached an agreement, and which defines the terms of their agreement. An honest, open exchange of accurate information is required. The contract should have the necessary level of detail to protect both parties and serve as a clear reference point should a dispute arise. Use your team of advisors to arrive at an equitable, final contract. Dollars spent early on will save you much heartache and grief later. Use your team to eliminate vague phrases which could later cost you money. There are no "standard contracts." Be sure the contract reflects your preferences and decisions. Do not sign anything having a "hold harmless" clause incorporated, since there is the very real possibility that you may pay monetary penalties arising from situations not under your control. Similarly, strike any clauses with the term *indemnify*! Your standard answer should be "Of course, I trust you, but my attorney does not trust you and insists on clear wording." Your advisory team should study how you are to be paid, and recommend the most favorable personal cash flow scenario from the outset. Especially important is attention to unforeseen events: for example, what would happen if the entity should declare bankruptcy? What is your responsibility to enrollees in that event? Also, who can change the fee schedule?

In some organizations, the primary care physician is responsible out of his own reimbursement for the inpatient and specialist costs incurred by enrollees assigned to him. There are, obviously, both monetary and legal considerations in reference to this arrangement. In the event of an enrollee having an untoward outcome, it may be alleged that you failed to make an appropriate referral to control costs. Likewise, what is your responsibility if there is a shortfall in hospitalization funds? Do you pay from your practice funds for any ordered outpatient tests or procedures?

Other considerations include the amount of notice you must provide before leaving the managed care plan. An area of provider concern, not found in a private office, is the possibility of an audit for quality of patient care or fraud. Beware of penalties and loss of any withheld payments for quality of care concerns. Obviously, there must be an appeals process, based on impartial review of facts, that is binding on you and the HMO. Similarly, who performs the inpatient review of patient care: a medical director, a registered nurse, or a non-medical person without the appropriate training or qualifications? Beware of transferable contracts. Does your contract specify your rights in the event that the HMO you joined is sold to another HMO?

Finally, is there a limit to the financial risk (stop-loss) you are subject to with each enrollee? For instance, one bone marrow transplant patient could wipe out a sizable portion of your annual hospitalization allotment. Spend adequate time with your team of consultants to discuss each aspect of the contract before final negotiation and signing. Check with those already in the plan to see if they advise any specific contract clarifications.

There are last minute items to review that may tip the balance if you are having difficulties in deciding between two potentially attractive but competing managed care plans. Visit all facilities in which you might potentially practice within the plan. What are the travel times? Is the administration supportive of providers? Query others who have exposure to the administration before deciding. What is the current financial position of the plan? What is the reputation of the plan in the community? Is enrollment in the plan increasing or decreasing? Are you being hired for a new position or a replacement position? If a replacement, find out who it is you are replacing and arrange for a candid conversation with that person. If such information is not forthcoming because the plan objects, be suspicious. Take a moment to find out if there is any impending state legislation that could adversely affect plan reimbursement. Finally, is employment stable in the region or are industrial lay-offs or closings imminent? (These could greatly decrease patient enrollment in the plan.)

The process of finding the right job in the right location cannot be left to chance. You should have your own team of consultants to advise you. A proper CV, in-depth interviews, leg work, questioning those in the know, and contract negotiation requires dedication, maturity, and diligent concentration on your part. You must understand the elements of a contract and be willing to prioritize your cash and noncash requirements to practice in a managed care environment. You must, in the final analysis, understand and accept the consequences of the contract you sign and live happily within its parameters.

MEDICAL MARKETING AND PRACTICE BUILDING

No matter what type of medical practice you decide upon, you must build your medical practice with referral sources and potential patients. Many physicians are uncomfortable with the term "marketing." Marketing yourself and your practice is an entirely different process from paid advertising. The term "marketing" is often misunderstood. Marketing is a social process by which individuals and groups obtain what they need and want through creating and exchanging ideas, products, services, and values with others. Physicians have been engaged in marketing themselves and their services for years without being aware of it. Your "market," as a new physician, includes patients, other physicians, employers, labor unions, government, schools, and the hospital(s). You must know the potential consumers of your services in order to be successful. You must define the type of practice you wish to have and meet the expectations of those you wish to serve.

Mentioned before in this chapter was the concept of a physician support team—attorney, accountant, insurance broker, and financial planner—that has the best interest of the physician as its focus. You may well wish to add to this team the services of a professional marketer. A coordinated plan of introduction to the community, provided within a defined budget, could be most efficiently developed with such guidance. The goal is to promote your services ethically to patients and referral sources. Who are you? What do you do? Where and when do you do it? What special procedures do you perform or what special skills do you possess? Schedule an office open house, and be sure everything is clean, neat, and orderly. Be sure to have printed take-away information for all who attend. Have separate handouts for professional and lay audiences with your office hours, address, and telephone numbers clearly indicated. Community leaders you should invite to your practice opening include educational leaders, corporate or industrial leaders, local medical society leaders, church and synagogue officials, officers of local service clubs, elected officials, and other influential community members recommended by friends and associates. Follow-up becomes key after the initial opening "blitz" of the community and its leaders. Be seen in your practice area. Join clubs, organizations, churches, special interest societies, hospital staffs and committees, and the county medical society. Offer to speak on subjects germane to your specialty and to write a column for the local newspaper, magazine, newsletter, or any circulated material. Arrange evening meals and lunches to get to know those who came to your open house, other medical colleagues, administrators, and community officials. Thank you notes to referring physicians, along with timely consultation notes, are mandatory. Thank you notes to anyone who refers patients are appreciated and are a thoughtful touch that will continue to build your practice. Again, consider a marketing consultant or a dedicated individual within your practice to organize and assist you in these efforts.

While many specialties operate by patient self-referral, some specialties are dependent on physician referrals. Study your patient flow. Where do your patients come from? Target these sources and decide on additional referral sources with good potential, then develop a plan to cultivate these sources. Prepare a short, suitable statement about yourself and your practice. On one page give all pertinent information about the practice, its location, hours, and telephone numbers. Then provide a short summary of your training and educational background. Finally, personalize yourself by describing your family, interests, and achievements. This summary can be used in a variety of forums such as a local paper, medical society bulletin, or health care magazine. It should be included with the invitations to the practice's opening party. Depending on the media type, include a photograph and CV. Similarly, print tasteful business cards and office stationery and foster the habit of passing out business cards and sending thank you notes for any worthwhile reason.

The following five step program has been suggested to market your practice. First, analyze the market. The local environment and the larger socioeconomic forces must be taken into consideration as they apply to your practice situation. Are you practicing state-of-the-art medicine? If not, get yourself up to date: learn the latest procedures and let colleagues and patients know of your new services. Is your office adequate, "patient-friendly," and suitable for existing patient volume and for additional patients? What types of patients are you serving? To add additional patients, can you draw from existing sources or will you need to develop new referral areas? Is the competition adding new physicians, services, space, satellite offices? If so, plan effective, well thought-out countermoves. Consider the impact of these largely unpredictable and uncontrollable socioeconomic forces on your practice:

1. Is the area you serve growing or declining in population and what is the median patient age?

2. What is the affordability of your services?
3. Is the area attracting new industry or is it dependent on a single, large employer?
4. Is there any environmental consideration that might affect your practice (medical conditions such as asthma from pollution)?
5. Are state or national political-legal considerations threatening your income, practice size, or imposing costly new regulations upon you?
6. Consider social and cultural issues affecting all local medical practices such as malpractice suits, charity care, uncompensated care, and rising numbers of AIDS and other types of cases.

Second, research and select the target market. Who do you want to be? What is your practice to be? What services do patients and employers want? What is lacking in the medical care provided in the community or region? Who are unserved or underserved patient groups?

Third, with the use of your marketing consultant or office staff, decide general marketing strategies. Can the office see more patients? Will you need more help? Would a satellite office better serve a portion of your patients? Do you need more room to offer new procedures and services? How can the office staff help this practice grow? Strategy is the development of an overall plan to accomplish goals.

Fourth, you must plan marketing tactics with your staff and team of consultants. Tactics are specific methods to assure a successful plan outcome.

Fifth and finally, get started! Modify the plan as you go. If a tactic works, stay with it. If not, discard it. Be goal oriented. Stay with your plan; modify your tactics and overall strategies to meet your goals. Develop meaningful monitors of your success such as numbers of new patients, increasing time to get an appointment, and increasing number of procedures. Tailor the effort devoted to this process to your circumstances, budget, and return on investment of personal time.

Some special considerations apply to building your practice through marketing. First and foremost, good marketing is no substitute for good medicine. You must be of good reputation, up-to-date on current practice and procedures, and a likable, open person. There is no substitute for this, although certain partners in a group practice may best represent the practice to colleagues, patients, and the public.

Second, be absolutely certain that all printed material that the practice distributes is accurate. Invite questions from recipients. Information should be useful, timely, understandable, and shared with others. Send colleagues articles pertinent to patients you have seen; they will learn from you and this will be appreciated. Always leave pertinent take-away materials with any civic or interest group you address. Be sure the materials are appropriate to that group. Put your name, telephone numbers, and address on all these materials. Speak only in the areas of your expertise and be prepared! When you volunteer for committees, health fairs, or organizations, find out what is expected of you. Be certain you have the site, the time, and the proper dress required for the occasion. Be seen where and in the light in which you wish to become known. Practice building is an ongoing process. Plan your tactics and strategies on an annual basis and have a budget and allotted time. The biggest failure of new practices is to forget to plan for ongoing promotion after the initial open house and practice promotion.

Finally, the hospitals you associate with may be willing to do shared promotions of procedures and services with you. Such an effort must result in a "win-win" situation for both your practice and the hospital. Be sure you and your consultant team have input into the process and can jointly shape the end product. The result must be tastefully presented and of real use to the target audience. Be certain you can deliver what is promised. Use available hospital data and do your homework before approaching the hospital administrator. Request advice from the hospital marketing staff and clearly specify what, if any, financial stake you have in the matter. Remember, the hospital will constantly be reevaluating its investment in you. They will want to see your admissions and your commitment to the institution on as many levels as possible.

CONSULTANT RELATIONS

As a practicing clinician, you will make referrals, receive referrals, or both. One of the earliest tests for the new physician is his or her performance as a consultant. Your colleagues will be watching closely how their patients are handled. The referring physician will want to be certain that the patient is returned to his practice and does not become your patient. Telephone the referring physician immediately after your consult. Present the differential diagnosis, suggested procedures or tests, and jointly develop an ongoing care plan. Follow up with a written thank you note for the consultation that includes the key elements of your discussion. Finally, a more formal written consultation note should follow. Maintain daily communication with the referring physician as long as you are on the case. Take every opportunity to teach the referring doctor about the medical condition for which you were consulted. If you are in a specialty role and the patient you are treating has no primary care physician, do not forget to recommend to the patient those physicians who refer to you. If you follow the outline above, your practice will certainly grow, and you will earn the respect and referrals of your colleagues.

There are a number of reasons to refer patients in your practice to specific specialists. Some patients need specialized testing or procedures requiring specialized physician skills. Patients with treatment failures or treatment dilemmas may require the specialist's input. Often, the patient or their family will request a consultation. They may have heard of a particular specialist for a specific problem. One example is teenagers seeking a dermatologic consult for acne. The family doctor, by referring such patients to the dermatologist, may lessen the patients' anxiety levels and may learn more about the treatment of the condition from the specialist's actions.

Encourage the patient and his family to join in the consultation process. Find the best possible consultant for the specific disease process. Let the patient know if there is clearly a best choice of consultant. Early on in a new practice, you will rely on the recommendations of your colleagues as to specialty referrals. With time and experience, you will use your own experience in picking consultants in whom you have the most confidence. Meet consultants face to face, talk with them, socialize with them. Go to continuing medical education presentations to learn new information and meet the presenters. If possible, assist at surgery and view the surgeon's techniques, his clinical knowledge of anatomy, and his judgment. Often, your own patients will be more comfortable if you are there to assist and view their problem first hand. Learn how readily available the consultant is to see your referrals. The situation should dictate the appropriate promptness of consultation. Be certain that your consultants understand that they will be getting all of your business, not just the patients with insurance.

As the referring physician, telephone your consultant as to why you are requesting his services. Establish the urgency of the consultation. Be clear as to whether the consultant is to assume the patient's care or only to make recommendations for further care. Put these instructions in writing and always forward copies of all pertinent patient medical records, tests, and reports. This way, expensive tests need not be repeated unless there is a change in the patient's condition. Recent studies have shown that the precise reason for consultation was not given in up to 22% of referrals. Since the consultant will likely be a stranger to your patient, you should prepare the patient as to what will take place, the time required, and additional tests or procedures that may be required. Inform the patient that while the consultant may provide some information directly to him, you are the patient's primary doctor and as such will take responsibility for thoroughly explaining the findings and what, if any, further medical intervention will be suggested.

As a consultant, you must clarify your role in patient care directly with the primary physician. When you request medical records, labs, and procedure reports, determine the urgency of the consult. Numerous studies document that communication of findings and recommendations to primary care physicians by specialists is often an area of failure. This is more common in university specialty clinics than with specialists in private practice. While the consultant's diagnosis and recommendations are most important, these recommendations are more likely to be followed when concise, specific, and relevant. There is a greater compliance rate if 5 or fewer recommendations are given. Give specific medication recommendations with dosages. Contingency plans formulated in advance are useful if the patient's condition worsens. Follow with a complete, dictated report after first telephoning the primary doctor and reaching a jointly agreed-upon initial treatment plan. Be sure that the dictated report you send can stand separately from the chart in the areas of patient history, physical findings, testing, differential diagnoses and final diagnosis, and treatment recommendations. At some point, your role in the patient's care is over. You should bow out gracefully, leaving the door open for further consultations as requested. Should the patient wish to leave his primary doctor and become your patient, usually the best course is to refuse to treat beyond the consultation. Your first loyalty is to your referring physicians. This is an ethical dilemma; you must not allow yourself to fall into this trap. Taking the long view, you will never see another patient from that referring doctor if you retain his or her patient.

There are some recommendations to insure that your first consultation is not your last. First, as discussed before, make your best effort to return the patient to the referring physician. The consultant must be firm and use persuasion and tact to direct the patient back to the referring physician. Second, clarify initially whether you are to mange the care of the patient or only make recommendations and suggestions. Further, if other consultants (specialists) are necessary for optimum patient care, will you, as consultant, select the specialist or will the primary care physician maintain control of this secondary referral?

Third, if the primary care physician is retaining control, be certain that the patient's family understand that you are seeing the patient only in consultation, and that the primary care physician has final patient care responsibility and will explain the patient's condition to the family. Fourth, review recommended tests and procedures with the referring physician prior to their performance, unless the procedure is required emergently. Physician to physician communication has no substitute and will eliminate misunderstanding and build good will. Fifth, try to make the consultation brief and to the point. Telephone calls are important and primary care physicians will appreciate them. Let the referring physicians know the reason for any delay in completing a consultation. Follow up with a concise, stand-alone consultation report in a timely fashion. Finally, unless the referring physician is clearly off base with regard to the consultation or procedure he is requesting of you, be supportive of the referring physician and teach him whatever you can about the patient's condition. If the referral was inappropriate, you must do what is right for the patient! However, you can do this with class and consideration for the primary care physician's feelings. Close adherence to these principles of consultation will insure your ongoing success in the face of an increasingly competitive medical practice market.

Chapter 12

Improving Interactions with Patients

GOAL

The goal of this chapter is to provide guidelines for improving your relationship with your patients.

GENERAL CONSIDERATIONS

The success of your practice is much more likely to depend upon the quality of your nonmedical interactions with patients than on the direct quality of medical care you provide for them. There are quite a number of considerations in improving relations with patients. Improved patient relations will directly benefit you in that it lessens your risk of being sued for malpractice, stimulates the flow of new referrals from satisfied patients to the practice, and makes the office a more pleasant and enjoyable place for everyone to work.

General considerations in improving relations with patients are mostly just common sense and courtesy. A good guide is to always treat the patient in your office as if he were a respected guest in your home. Even though you might not spend much time with the patient on an office visit, you should avoid giving the impression that you are hurried or harassed. Taking the brief time to assume a comfortable posture when you talk to the patient, avoiding performance of other paperwork during the patient exam and visit, and facing the patient when talking to him all give the patient a sense that you are devoting your full attention to him during his visit.

Most patients appreciate being asked small niceties such as questions about their family members, hobbies, or social activities. As part of your medical charting system, it may be helpful to note specific items of personal information about the patient (such as names of immediate family members, hobbies, travel experiences, military experiences) at a prominent point in the patient's chart, so that you could quickly refer to this when beginning your visit with the patient. At some point in the patient visit, making physical contact with the patient actually serves as a significant reassurance to the patient. This could include feeling a wrist pulse briefly, listening briefly to the chest, or patting the patient's shoulder. Even when these particular things are not absolutely required for patient examination, most patients still find some bit of direct contact desirable and reassuring. They may feel short shifted in their visit if this does not occur.

SPECIFIC CONSIDERATIONS

Here are more specific things to consider doing that are usually greatly appreciated by patients.

1. Send get well cards and/or flowers to your patients who are significantly ill or hospitalized.
2. Send thank you notes to patients who refer other new patients to you or who otherwise help to publicize your practice.
3. Call patients to see how they are doing the day after an office visit for a significant problem or a day or so after their discharge from the hospital (unless they are scheduled for an early post-hospitalization office visit with you).
4. Send birthday cards, anniversary cards, and/or holiday cards to your patients regularly.
5. Include brief patient education sheets, brochures, or information about your new medical procedures with other routine communications to patients (such as monthly mailed bills or recall notices for follow-up visits).
6. Take the time to appropriately educate patients about their conditions and medications. While at first this may seem to take excessive time, in the long run it will usually save you a lot of follow-up phone calls from patients for clarification of their instructions or effects of medications.
7. Carefully construct written discharge instructions for patients seen in the office. There are a number of software packages of discharge instructions available which can be readily modified to suit your individual style of practice.

8. Some patients find it most helpful to receive a detailed schedule of the times to take their medications, with dosages and names of the medications clearly noted. Providing patients with a reduced-size copy of their electrocardiogram (especially if they have baseline electrocardiographic abnormalities) can be invaluable in case of an emergency. Patients should be encouraged to carry these documents with them at all times.
9. Encourage patients with a chronic medical problem to obtain a Medic Alert bracelet or necklace. These are currently available starting at $25 and are obtainable by calling 1–800–432–5378 or writing Medic Alert, 2323 Colorado Avenue, Turlock, CA 95380. Medic Alert has informational brochures about the value of this program which may be useful to post in your waiting room. Certainly, Medic Alert registration should be strongly encouraged for all patients with insulin-dependent diabetes, cardiac and seizure disorders, or recurrent syncope.
10. Reading materials, such as magazines or brochures, should be available in the exam rooms as well as in the waiting room so as to make the time pass more quickly for patients awaiting exam or test results.
11. If your practice serves two different groups of patients or patients of different ages, you should consider having more than one television for use in the waiting areas. One television could be kept tuned to channels with children's programs to serve the pediatric patients in the waiting room, whereas another could be tuned to a news channel or other adult-oriented program. If the television were connected to a VCR, then videotapes (either of entertainment programs or patient education programs) could be run continuously. It would actually be fairly easy to construct your own videotape for use in the waiting room, describing the practice or showing you personally presenting patient education information in a conversational or lecture-like format.
12. Dispense sample medication from your office whenever possible. Patients greatly appreciate this service as it spares them having to go directly from the office to a pharmacy to obtain their prescription on the day of the visit. By giving a few sample doses of medication, the patient has much more flexibility in getting to the pharmacy to obtain the complete prescription. In addition, if you are seeing patients late in the day and the local pharmacies all close at about that same time,

the patient would not be able to get the prescription filled after leaving the office. Sample medications in this situation are especially useful. In addition, having a supply of sample medications in the office allows you to selectively give patients who cannot afford certain medications a course of drug treatment at no cost to them. If you utilize any sample medications of narcotics or benzodiazepines, be certain to keep dispensing records on them and keep access to them restricted as for other DEA-scheduled drugs.

13. Whenever possible, maintain office hours that are convenient for your patient population. This usually entails having evening office hours at least one evening a week. This would allow people that have 9–5 jobs Monday through Friday to make an office visit without having to take time off from work; it would also allow parents to bring in children after school.
14. It is important to avoid any ingestion of alcoholic drinks prior to seeing patients in the office or making house calls or hospital visits. Even though one or two drinks may not impair one's medical ability or performance, just the odor of alcohol on your breath might significantly upset a patient or family member.

PATIENT QUESTIONNAIRE

At intervals in your practice, it would be helpful to utilize a patient questionnaire to determine the patients' perceptions of how well you and your practice are doing. You should structure the questionnaire to address questions you feel are important to the practice or things that you would potentially change, depending on patient feedback. Sample questionnaires are available from the American Society of Internal Medicine and the American Medical Association (see the reference list for this chapter). Questionnaires could be given to patients as they are waiting for exam or as they are being discharged from the office. An anonymous drop box could be used to return forms. Alternatively, the patients could be provided with self-addressed, stamped envelopes in which to return the questionnaires to the office. Items to consider addressing in the questionnaire are the patient's perception of waiting times; problems with access to the practice; patient's perception of quality of care offered; evaluation of the attitudes and helpfulness of the office staff; ease of compliance with the billing and other office paperwork procedures; and additional services that should be offered by the practice. Questionnaires for patients should be structured to allow specific choices as answers for each question rather than vague open-ended answers. Options of "do not know" or "no opinion" should be included as a possible response to each question. Topics that would embarrass the patient or would require medical training for response should be avoided.

WRITTEN COMMUNICATIONS TO PATIENTS

An excellent way to establish a good relationship with each new patient is to utilize a well-written "welcome to the practice" letter. This should be mailed to each new patient before the first office visit or given to the patient at their first visit in the office. General topics to be addressed in the welcome letter include the following:

1. Office hours and days of the week
2. Procedure for scheduling appointments
3. Types of problems or conditions seen in the office
4. Fee schedule and methods of payment
5. Guidelines for HMO and PPO patients
6. How telephone calls are handled by the office
7. Type of personnel who will respond to phone calls, and the procedure for routing phone calls after hours
8. Interaction with other physicians
9. Other specifics related to the type of practice

In addition to the "welcome to the practice" letter, it is very helpful to have a patient information booklet and/or a periodic patient newsletter to disseminate information about the practice. A patient information booklet could be fairly expensive to produce, depending on its length and use of photographs or pictures. The patient information booklet should be very carefully written to avoid having it become quickly outdated, thereby necessitating frequent revisions. Basically, the patient information booklet would be an expanded source of information about the practice compared to the "welcome to the practice" letter. If properly written, it could also be distributed as an information source about the practice to potential referral physicians. Items to consider addressing in the patient information booklet are the following:

1. The physician's general philosophy of practice and relationship to other health care professionals
2. Personal and training background information on each member of the practice (including educational background, additional specialty training programs completed, certifications, brief relevant family and personal history perhaps including hobbies and special interests)
3. Services provided by the practice
   A. Emergency versus routine scheduled exams and treatments
   B. Age range and other restrictions on types of patients seen
   C. Types of medical problems dealt with in the practice
   D. Procedures or additional technical services offered by the practice
   E. Additional occupational medicine or business services offered by the practice
4. Billing and payment policies and procedures
5. Relationship of the practice to hospitals and other health care organizations
6. How emergencies of different types are handled in the practice

Use of a periodic newsletter for patients in your practice can be very helpful in promoting the practice as well as improving patient care. You could utilize the newsletter to simply present educational information on health care in general or on self care and preventive medicine. Additionally, you could present material that would actually encourage patients to come in to the office to be checked for certain symptoms or problems or for follow-up care for known chronic problems. You could also utilize a newsletter to correct sensationalized misinformation presented by the mass media. Easily and quickly obtainable sources for patient health care information include discharge instruction sheets from your local emergency department or from one of the commercially available computerized discharge information systems such as LogiCare.

Chapter 13

Enjoying Your Practice

GOAL

The goal of this chapter is to present some general guidelines on getting enjoyment from your medical career.

INTRODUCTION

It is important to keep a proper perspective on how rewarding a career in private medical practice can be. Because of the unpreventable or self-induced nature of most human illness, there will always be a need for medical care by physicians. The demand for physicians is essentially independent of economic recession and other societal problems, although it may actually be increased by such problems as drug abuse and trauma due to violent behavior. Despite the alleged physician surplus in this country, a quick look at the "jobs available" section in the back of any medical journal will demonstrate that there are a large number of medical positions open in all specialties and in all sections of the country. Even with the current trend of increasing government interference with private practice medicine, it will undoubtedly continue to be true that private practice physicians will earn high incomes and have an overall degree of job security greater than almost any other profession. What follows are some general guidelines that may help you to maintain enjoyment of your medical practice.

DO NOT NEGLECT YOUR FAMILY

Although the practice of medicine to some extent always demands putting the care of the patient first, you should make every effort to structure your life so that your family is not neglected. This is probably the most difficult aspect of one's personal life to regulate when in private medical practice. For very important family milestones (anniversaries, music recitals, graduations, etc.) try to arrange to be totally "off" that day, with your practice fully covered by someone else. Each week you should make a point of devoting some specific time directly to family activities.

DO NOT BE AFRAID TO TAKE VACATIONS

If your finances permit, you should take vacation time by traveling away from the community in which your medical practice is located. If you stay in the local area for your vacation, there is a tendency to spend that time answering medical phone calls or dealing with other aspects of your practice. Vacation time should be essentially 100% separated from medical practice work time. Scheduling several one-week vacations during the year rather than one much longer three- or four-week vacation is usually less disruptive to a medical practice; however, certain types of desirable vacations cannot be squeezed into a week.

If the members of your family have different interests, consider arranging the vacation to spend one day at an activity preferred by one family member, the next day at an activity preferred by another family member, and then the third day at an activity you most enjoy. Repeat this cycle for the remainder of the vacation. This way everyone in the family will be able to have at least a portion of the vacation doing what he or she enjoys most. In general, you should not do any concentrated continuing medical education activity on your vacation, although some light, occasional reading of medical journals is not unreasonable. Combining a vacation with a continuing medical education conference can be successful, but you need to be sure that there are activities during the conference period that you can participate in with the family rather than spending all your time separately at medical conference sessions. Better yet, plan to spend your vacation a few days before or after the conference.

MAINTAIN YOUR OWN HEALTH

Obviously, if you avoid smoking, excess alcohol consumption, and overeating, it will make it much easier for you to nonhypocritically recommend these important health care measures to your patients. Your patients will realize you "practice what you preach." On days when you will be working in the office, you should take the time to have an adequate breakfast and lunch.

Proper food intake will help you maintain your efficiency and ability to work at a demanding pace. Despite the demands of your practice, you should set aside specific times each week for regular exercise and not allow nonemergent practice concerns to interfere with this scheduled exercise time.

MAINTAIN A PATTERN OF SELF-EDUCATION

This consideration is perhaps the easiest to fulfill as it is essentially mandated by most states' continuing medical education requirements for maintenance of a medical license. Your patients will have greater respect for you as they realize you are keeping up with medical developments and utilizing new proven medical treatments. You can and should take pride in keeping up with medical developments. Even attending seminars or reading materials outside your own specialty can be useful, especially in improving your interactions with consultants.

DEVELOP SOME HOBBIES

Physicians who have devoted their entire lives only to medical practice and have never developed any hobbies or interests outside of medicine can experience extreme depression on retiring from practice. To avoid this potential disaster, it is important to develop interests and activities outside of medicine. The authors strongly recommend having an interest in at least one outdoor hobby and one indoor hobby (so that you have something fun to do regardless of the weather). The list of potential hobbies and activities is, of course, huge and so dependent upon one's personal interests that the authors will not attempt to make any specific recommendations here. The ideal situation is to choose hobbies in which other family members are interested so that their participation in the hobby makes it an enjoyable family activity. From a self-interest point of view, participation in some hobbies may increase your contact with persons who might then become new patients in your practice or refer patients to your practice.

GET INVOLVED IN YOUR COMMUNITY

As a physician you occupy an almost automatic leadership position within the community and your knowledge and advice tend to be respected immediately. By participating in various community organizations, you would also, of course, increase your exposure to the community and thereby might increase your practice referrals. Involvement with community groups would also allow you to promote important aspects of health education and preventive medicine. Many local organizations like to have a physician as a dinner speaker for their organization's meetings. You might even develop an interest in pursuing politics as a sideline to your medical career. Physicians are among the more fortunate people in society. Educated, experienced, and economically well-off, we have an obligation to do more for those we live among than just practice medicine. Churches, schools, community organizations, music and art groups, scouting, and local government all appreciate our involvement.

DO NOT ISOLATE YOURSELF FROM OTHER MEDICAL PROFESSIONALS

Even if you have a nonhospital-based practice or do not have hospital admission privileges, it is very important to maintain regular contact with other medical professionals, especially within your own community. This can act as a source for further referrals to your practice, as well as a source for continuing medical education. By maintaining these contacts, you may also utilize them for informal advice for difficult-to-handle cases.

Another consideration is to develop a relationship with various medical education institutions. Having students (medical students, physical therapy students, paramedics, etc.) visit your office practice or see patients with you in the office can be a very rewarding experience. This allows you to act as a role model for these students, as well as a means for you to encourage people to pursue a career in practice situations similar to your own. It may also allow you to cultivate future partners for the practice. The main reward, however, is more often just having the stimulation of contact with younger people in training. The major consideration is to verify that there is malpractice insurance coverage for the student while involved in your practice (if the student is to be doing any patient care). Malpractice coverage is usually provided by the student's teaching institution, but under certain circumstances you might need to alter your own malpractice policy to cover the student's activities within your office. For many medical specialties, there is currently a trend toward more involvement with outpatient, office-based care; thus, there is a need for more office-based training sites. This would apply to medical schools and physical therapy schools as well as pediatric, family practice, and internal medicine residency programs.

BE TOLERANT OF YOUR COLLEAGUES

They, like you, try to do the right thing. Sometimes, of course, despite the best efforts, things just do not go well. Everyone of us has made mistakes. If you have concerns about another practitioner's management of a patient's problem, call and talk it over. Often you will find the other professional is well-informed, made a reasonable decision under the circumstances, and does not resent, but appreciates, discussing the situation with you.

ENJOY AND RESPECT YOUR EMPLOYEES

Be kind, tolerant, understanding, and fair. Your life will benefit immeasurably. You set the tone of your practice—others follow, up or down.

ENJOY YOUR PATIENTS!

They are often interesting, humorous, insightful, and almost always have a vocation different from yours. Treat them as you would want to be treated yourself. See them on time. Their time is valuable too! Timeliness is a gesture of respect that patients notice. Don't hesitate to go the extra mile. Such acts are not forgotten, and your satisfaction with medical practice will be enhanced.

Suggested Readings

General

Fox YM. "Going into Practice" column in *Resident and Staff Physician.* For a number of years, Ms. Fox has written at least one article every month in the journal *Resident and Staff Physician.* She also answers questions about private practice from letters sent to the journal (80 Shore Road, Port Washington, NY 11050). Ms. Fox is an experienced practice management consultant from California. Her articles cover the entire range of topics relevant to private medical practice; they are well-written and full of very practical advice. Her articles address each of the specific chapter topics in this book.

Gitnick G, Rothenberg F, Weiner JL. *The Business of Medicine.* New York: Elsevier Science Publishing Inc., 1991, 526 pp. Detailed. Includes chapters on adding a partner, practice mergers, coping with stress and burnout, selling or dissolving a practice, and retirement.

Henderson-Damon, C, ed. *The Business Side of Medical Practice.* American Medical Association, 1989, 155 pp. One of the AMA's Practice Development Services publications. Well-written and detailed. Lacks information on office design and layout. The AMA has a large number of practice development brochures, booklets, book, videotapes, etc. For current prices and ordering information call 1–800–621–8335.

Szostak-Ricardo, M. *The New Practice Handbook.* New York: McGraw-Hill Inc., 1991, 166 pp. Has useful tables, charts, and sample forms.

Chapter 1

Fulton, Longshore, and Associates, Inc.: Choosing the right job in the best market. *Hospital Physician* 1992;(May):48–59.

Kalogredis VJ: *Practice Options for Today's Young Physician.* Harrisburg: Pennsylvania Medical Society, 1989, 26 pp. Brief overview, but provides good framework for general career planning.

Kelly N: Volunteering overseas. *Hospital Physician* 1991;(December):49–52.

Reeves DD: Careers in the U.S. Air Force. *Hospital Physician* 1992;(May):64–71.

Trenz PR: Defining your career objectives. *Hospital Physician* 1985;(May):15–17.

Chapter 2

Fox YM: Where is your specialty needed? *Res Staff Physician* 1987;33(11):127–139. Has good reference list of addresses of specialty organizations.

Share SH, Sweeney DR: Selecting the best private office location. *Hospital Physician* 1985;(November):34–40.

Chapter 3

Anonymous: How to prepare your curriculum vitae. *Res Staff Physician* 1987;33(4):143–148.

Fox YM: How to present at an interview. *Res Staff Physician* 1988; 34(10):119–123.

Fulton AA: The endgame: The interview process and the evaluation of offers. *Hospital Physician* 1991;(December):38–42.

Mack SC: Practice basics: Resumes that produce jobs. *Hospital Physician* 1991;(March):12–16.

Chapter 4

Auclair RA, Dallabrida D: Restrictive covenants in physician employment agreements. *Penn Med* 1992;(November):16–19.

Fox YM: What to expect if you are recruited by a hospital. *Res Staff Physician* 1987;33(2):104–108.

Fox YM: How to negotiate a contract. *Res Staff Physician* 1987;33(4): 123–125.

Fox YM: How to evaluate a job offer. *Res Staff Physician* 1988;34(12): 133–127.

Pennsylvania Medical Society Council on Medical Practice. *Planning for Your Retirement.* Harrisburg: Pennsylvania Medical Society, 1986, 41 pp. Has sample forms and contracts.

Robinson R: A primer on how to analyze contracts and avoid the traps. *Consultant* 1988;28(7):74–77.

Stuart JG: Negotiating a group-practice contract: The physician's checklist. *Hospital Physician* 1992;(February):59–64.

Vipond J, Musselman J: *A Physician's Guide to Employment Contracts.* Harrisburg: Pennsylvania Medical Society, 1991, 74 pp.

Chapter 5

American Medical Association: *Optimum Timetable for Starting Your Practice.* 1989, 20 pp.

American Medical Association. *U.S. Medical Licensure Statistics and Current Licensure Requirements, 1992 Edition.* (Publication OP-399091).

Fox YM: Timetable for starting your practice. *Res Staff Physician* 1991; 37(8):83–84.

Fox YM: How to obtain hospital privileges. *Res Staff Physician* 1991; 37(12):75–78.

Lang DA: The medical staff is on your side. *Res Staff Physician* 1987; 33(13):97–100.

Chapter 6

American Medical Association: *Planning Guide for Physician's Medical Facilities.* 1979, 35 pp. Nicely detailed; has a number of sample floor plan diagrams.

Fox YM: Should you have a lab in your office? *Res Staff Physician* 1990; 36(6):59–62.

Fox YM: Ordering supplies and controlling inventory. *Res Staff Physician* 1990;36(10):108–112.

Fox YM: Equipment needed to start a practice. *Res Staff Physician* 1990; 36(11):83–88.

Fox YM: How to design your office. *Res Staff Physician* 1992;38(5):179–181.

Kroger JS: The office laboratory—A boon to your practice? Or a burden? *Consultant* 1987; 27(5):70–73.

Ricardo M: The physical facility. In *The New Practice Handbook,* pp. 38–47. New York: McGraw-Hill Inc, 1991.

Terribilini CJ: The Americans with Disabilities Act. *J Emerg Med Serv* 1992;(July):63–69.

Chapter 7

American Medical Association. *Valuing a Medical Practice.* 1989, 8 pp.

American Medical Association. *Buying and Selling Medical Practices: A Valuation Guide.* 1989, 100 pp.

American Medical Association. *Financing a Practice: Start-up, Acquisition, or Expansion.* 1991, 56 pp.

Fox YM: How to share office space. *Res Staff Physician* 1991;37(4):73–77.

Fox YM: How to obtain a loan to start a practice. *Res Staff Physician* 1992;38(2):157–160.

Fox YM: Leasing space: Definitions and guidelines. *Res Staff Physician* 1992;38(4):131–134.

Chapter 8

American Medical Association. *Risk Management Principles and Commentaries for the Medical Office.* 1990, 31 pp.

Anders GT, Smith PW: The new OSHA regulations. *Penn Med* April 1992 (Suppl):A1–A4.

Fox YM: How many employees do you need to start a practice? *Res Staff Physician* 1985;31(12):31–35.

Fox YM: How to prevent embezzlement in your office. *Res Staff Physician* 1990;36(8):67–76.

Fox YM: How to hire an efficient staff. *Res Staff Physician* 1992;38(8):85–87.

Fox YM: How to be an effective employer. *Res Staff Physician* 1992; 38(9):108–112.

Fox YM: How to fire an employee. *Res Staff Physician* 1992;38(10):91–97.

Chapter 9

American Medical Association. *Medicolegal Forms with Legal Analysis.* Contains over 80 sample forms.

Fox YM: How to keep your finger on the financial pulse of your practice. *Res Staff Physician* 1986;32(10):75–81.

Fox YM: Patient flow and scheduling. *Res Staff Physician* 1990;36(4):93–98.

Fox YM: Forms needed in a private practice. *Res Staff Physician* 1990; 36(5):151–153.

Fox YM: How to establish and keep medical records. *Res Staff Physician* 1991;37(5):137–140.

Fox YM: How to set your fees. *Res Staff Physician* 1992;38(3):147–153.

Fox YM: Basic principles of bookkeeping. *Res Staff Physician* 1992; 38(11):73–78.

Johnson DM: Improving recordkeeping: A filing system that works. *Hospital Physician* 1985;(July):70–71.

Chapter 10

Kasten GW: What you need to know about financial planners. *Res Staff Physician* 1989;35(1):125–128.

Kasten GW: Financial planning basics. *Res Staff Physician* 1990;36(1): 116–118.

Kasten GW: What you need to know about retirement plans. *Res Staff Physician* 1992;38(2):151–153.

Chapter 11

Barnett B, Waxman JM: HMO reimbursement and the noncontracted physician. *Medical Interface* 1992;(September):45–47.

Boren SD: The four types of health maintenance organizations. *Res Staff Physician* 1991;37(11):105–106.

Boren SD: What HMO's do with their money. *Res Staff Physician* 1992; 38(4):141–142.

Fox YM: Going into practice. *Res Staff Physician* 1987;33(9):107–108.

Chapter 12

Aluise JJ: How to promote health awareness and your practice simultaneously. *Consultant* 1991;(December):33–45.

American Medical Association. *Patient Survey Questionnaire.* (Publication OP-121).

Fox YM: How to cement the physician-patient relationship. *Res Staff Physician* 1990;36(12):59–68.

Fox YM: Preventing frivolous malpractice claims. *Res Staff Physician* 1991;37(2):77–83.

McDonell TH: How to survive in a doctor surplus. *Res Staff Physician* 1987;33(7):113–119.

Yenney SL: *Marketing Your Internal Medicine Practice: A Practical Guide for Internists and Their Staffs.* Washington, DC: American Society of Internal Medicine, 1988.

Yenney SL: How to survey patients and staff to improve your practice. *Consultant* 1989;(December):41–52.

Chapter 13

Pfifferling J: Things I wish they taught in medical school. *Res Staff Physician* 1990;36(4):85–92.

Roberts WC: Words to the wise. *Res Staff Physician* 1986;32(9):107–108.

References Concerning Compliance With the Americans With Disabilities Act

1. Equal Employment Opportunity Commission
   1801 L Street, NW
   Washington, DC 20507
   202–663–4900
   (For concerns about disabled employee hiring)

2. Department of Justice
   Office of Americans with Disabilities Act
   Civil Rights Division
   P.O. Box 66118
   Washington, DC 20035–6118
   202–514–0301
   (For concerns about public access for the disabled)

3. Disability and Business Technical Assistance Center
   1–800–949–4232
   or National Rehabilitation Hospital ADA Compliance Program
   102 Irving Street, NW
   Washington, DC 10010
   202–877–1947
   (For technical assistance on compliance with the ADA)

4. Architectural and Transportation Barriers Compliance Board
   1111 18th Street, NW, Suite 501
   Washington, DC 10036
   1–800–872–2253
   (For information on accessibility design in construction)

5. Department of Transportation
   400 Seventh Street, SW
   Washington, DC 20590
   202–366–9305
   (For concerns about ADA requirements affecting transport)

6. Federal Communications Commission
   1919 M Street, NW
   Washington, DC 20554
   202–623–7260
   (For concerns about ADA requirements for language translation)

Appendix B

Sample companies from whom to obtain catalogs from which to order: (NOTE: These are included for reference only and not as an endorsement.)

1. James Limited
   2412 West North Avenue
   Chicago, IL 60647
   1–800–James Ltd
   FAX 312–486–6596 (all types of office equipment, furniture and supplies, as well as medical supplies)
2. Colwell Systems, Inc.
   201 Kenyon Road
   P.O. Box 9024
   Champaign, IL 61826–9024
   1–800–637–1140 (in Illinois 1–800–252–6960)
   (office forms and paperwork; customized paper materials)
3. IDE Interstate Medical Supply Catalogue
   1500 New Horizons Boulevard
   Amityville, NY 11701
   1–800–666–8100
   FAX 526–957–1678 (wholesale pharmaceuticals, medical supplies and equipment, business office supplies and equipment)
4. Medical Arts Press
   3440 Winnetka Avenue, North
   Minneapolis, MN 55427–2093
   1–800–328–2179 (in Minnesota call collect 612–545–3200)
   (office supplies and paperwork)
5. R & J Medical Supply, Inc.
   7940 North 81 Street
   Milwaukee, WI 53223
   1–800–992–5668
   FAX 414–355–3975 (medical supplies)
6. Pharmaceutical Discounters, Inc.
   488 Gwinnett Drive
   Lawrenceville, GA 30245
   1–800–933–3903
   (wholesale pharmaceuticals)

7. Intercity EMS
   Emergency Medical Supplies, Inc.
   841 McDonald Avenue
   Brooklyn, NY 11218
   1–800–468–7289
   FAX 718–436–8806
8. Medibadge
   P.O. Box 12456
   Omaha, NB 68112
   1–800–228–0040
   (stickers and other items for pediatric patients and customized office announcement materials)
9. Associated Medical Products
   400 West Boden Street
   Milwaukee, WI 53207–7120
   1–800–926–6100
   FAX 1–800–926–4610

A further listing of companies can be obtained from:

10. Health Industry Distributors Associates
    1701 Pennsylvania Avenue, NW
    Washington, DC 10006

Appendix C

Complying With the OSHA Regulations for Occupational Exposure to Blood or Other Potentially Infectious Materials

The Occupational Safety and Health Administration (OSHA) has developed regulations that took effect in 1992 requiring compliance by private medical practices for protection of their employees from potentially infectious materials. These regulations apply to almost all private medical practices except those which are unincorporated and have no nonphysician staff. OSHA basically requires all physician employers to comply with the regulations with the aim to protect the employees who might come into "occupational exposure with potentially infectious materials such as blood or other body fluids." The regulations include the following basic requirements:

1. Identify the staff members who may have a potential risk of exposure;
2. Provide resources and equipment for protection of the staff;
3. Develop specific work routines to lessen the chances of infection;
4. Have a written plan to limit exposures by the office staff;
5. Maintain written records documenting staff training and on the vaccination status of the staff.

Because any office staff member who might even occasionally have to clean up spilled body fluids (such as emesis) would have a "potential exposure," the physician employer might want to rewrite the job duties of that position to exclude that kind of activity. Specific features of the OSHA regulations include the following requirements:

1. Training about biohazard avoidance and treatment of potential exposures must be formally conducted. Training sessions must provide office staff with a copy of the OSHA regulations and general medical explanation of the risks of and specific diseases caused by body fluid contact or transmission. Further, the proper selection, use, and disposal of protective devices and the equipment must be reviewed. The procedures to be routinely followed in the office for exposure incidents must be explained, and information on hepatitis B vaccination (which must be provided by the practice free of charge to the office staff who may have the exposures) is necessary. Usually, an extensive office training manual will need to be written to assure that all these requirements are met and to enable all employees to have access to the same information and training program.
2. Extensive recordkeeping of both exposure incidents as well as a training record for each employee must be maintained. Records of each occupational exposure must be kept until 30 years after termination of employment. Records of employee training must be kept for at least 3 years following the date of the training.
3. Staff must be provided with appropriate personal protective equipment and instruction on its proper use. This would include gloves, nonpermeable gowns, coats, face shields, mouthpieces, and possibly ventilation devices (such as pocket mask or S-tube with one-way valve). The employer physician is mandated by the regulations to verify that the employees are actually using the protective devices appropriately. The employer is subject to OSHA sanctions if an employee does not properly use protective devices, and the employee, himself, even though at fault, is not really liable.
4. Used hypodermic needles or other needles used in contact with patient blood or tissue may not be bent, recapped, sheared, or broken. Needles must be disposed of in puncture-resistant and leak-proof containers labeled with a standard biohazard symbol. Broken metal or glass pieces must

not be cleaned up by hand but instead cleaned up with brushes or other mechanical items.

5. Hand-washing facilities must be easily available in all parts of the office where exposures may occur. The physician employer is responsible for ensuring that employees actually perform hand washing after each potential contact with infectious material.
6. Specific cleaning and decontamination procedures must be followed for each potential spill or environmental contamination with body fluids.
7. All potentially contaminated laundry must be placed in leak proof containers denoted by a biohazard symbol. Office staff are not allowed to take contaminated laundry home for cleaning. The office practice must either have a contract with a commercial laundry or have appropriate laundry facilities in the office to clean all contaminated laundry safely. Additional procedures must be followed in the event of a potentially significant body fluid exposure by an employee.

These procedures will vary significantly by state because state laws governing drawing blood from and notifying potentially infected source patients vary considerably. In a number of states this proper sequence would be as follows:

1. Document the circumstances and cause of the exposure by the employee;
2. Identify the person who was the source of the potentially infectious material;
3. Obtain the employee's consent for testing the employee's blood for viral antigens or antibodies;
4. Obtain consent and test the source person's blood for viral antigen or antibodies, if the employee's results were negative;
5. Make available appropriate counseling and postexposure medical precautions for both the employee and the source person.

Index

Page numbers in *italics* denote figures; those followed by "t" denote tables.